Workbook for Surgical Technology:
Principles and Practice

Sixth Edition

Prepared by:

Julie Armistead, CST, CRCST, BA
Surgical Technology Program Director
Virginia College
Macon, Georgia

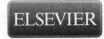

3251 Riverport Lane
St. Louis, Missouri 63043

WORKBOOK FOR SURGICAL TECHNOLOGY: PRINCIPLES AND
PRACTICE, SIXTH EDITION

ISBN: 978-0-323-35417-2

Notices

Knowledge and best practice in this field are constantly changing. As new research and experience broaden
our understanding, changes in research methods, professional practices, or medical treatment may become
necessary.

Practitioners and researchers must always rely on their own experience and knowledge in evaluating and
using any information, methods, compounds, or experiments described herein. In using such information or
methods they should be mindful of their own safety and the safety of others, including parties for whom they
have a professional responsibility.

With respect to any drug or pharmaceutical products identified, readers are advised to check the most
current information provided (i) on procedures featured or (ii) by the manufacturer of each product to be
administered, to verify the recommended dose or formula, the method and duration of administration, and
contraindications. It is the responsibility of practitioners, relying on their own experience and knowledge
of their patients, to make diagnoses, to determine dosages and the best treatment for each individual
patient, and to take all appropriate safety precautions.

To the fullest extent of the law, neither the Publisher nor the authors, contributors, or editors, assume any
liability for any injury and/or damage to persons or property as a matter of products liability, negligence or
otherwise, or from any use or operation of any methods, products, instructions, or ideas contained in the
material herein.

Vice President and Publisher: Andrew Allen
Executive Content Strategist: Jennifer Janson
Senior Content Development Specialist: Kelly Brinkman
Publishing Services Manager: Catherine Jackson
Project Manager: Kiruthiga Kasthuriswamy

Printed in United States

Last digit is the print number: 9 8 7 6 5 4 3 2 1

Preface

The goal of this workbook is to help students apply and master key concepts and skills presented in *Surgical Technology: Principles and Practice, sixth edition.* The exercises in this workbook will reinforce comprehension of material from the textbook.

The following exercises will provide a sufficient review of concepts and will allow the student to apply the concepts from the text:

- Each chapter begins with a *key term* review. A list of important terms in the corresponding book chapter is provided to test student comprehension of main concepts.
- **Short Answer** response questions apply knowledge learned from the text to a variety of situations.
- A variety of question formats test knowledge of concepts in the book, including **matching** and **multiple choice**.
- **Labelling** exercises reinforce important anatomy concepts a surgical technologist should be familiar with.
- **Case Studies** provide the practical skills of being a surgical technologist. Patient scenarios allow students to be familiar with real-life situations that will prepare them for the job.

Best wishes as you begin your journey to become a surgical technologist!

Contents

1 The Surgical Technologist

Student's Name _____

KEY TERMS

Write the definition for each term.

1. ABHES: _____

2. ACS: _____

3. Allied health profession: _____

4. AMA: _____

5. ANSI: _____

6. AORN: _____

7. ARC/STSA: _____

8. Assistant circulator: _____

9. AST: _____

10. CAAHEP: _____

11. Certification: _____

12. Continuing education: _____

13. CST: _____

14. CST-CFA: _____

15. Licensure: _____

16. National Certifying Examination for Surgical Technologist: _____

17. NBSTSA: _____

18. NCCT: _____

19. Nonsterile team members: _____

20. ORT: _____

21. Professional attributes: _____

22. Proprietary school: _____

23. Scrub: _____

24. Sterile personnel: _____

25. Surgical conscience: _____

SHORT ANSWERS

Provide a short answer for each question or statement.

1. What are the differences between the titles TS-C and CST?

   _____

   _____

2. What is the ARC/STSA, and what is its role?

   _____

   _____

3. What are the educational options for students who want to be surgical technologists?

   _____

   _____

4. Why is it important for a practicing surgical technologist to engage in continued education?

   _____

   _____

5. Name three areas of potential employment for a graduate surgical technologist.

   _____

   _____

6. What are the minimum requirements for an educator position?

   _____

   _____

7. What is the difference between a surgical educator and a surgical clinical preceptor?

_____

_____

8. What is the difference between ABHES and CAAHEP?

_____

_____

9. Why must a surgical technologist have good organizational skills?

_____

_____

10. Why does the AST organization need or want to work on legislative actions?

_____

_____

11. What are the educational requirements for a surgical technologist to become a surgical first assistant?

_____

_____

12. How did the field of surgical technology become what it is today?

_____

_____

MATCHING

Match the following individuals with a description of their roles. Individuals may have multiple roles, and each question may have more than one answer.

_____ 1. Maintain retraction of tissue

_____ 2. Scrub, gown, and glove self and team members

_____ 3. Communicate effectively with surgeon to prevent errors.

_____ 4. Nonsterile team member who assists the sterile surgical team

_____ 5. Performs surgical maneuvers such as cutting tissue, maintaining hemostasis, and suturing under the direction of the primary surgeon.

_____ 6. Specialist in the preparation, handling, and use of instruments

_____ 7. Prepares drugs and solutions for use in the surgical wound.

_____ 8. Teaches others in surgery

_____ 9. Pursues an advanced degree in hospital administration and management

_____ 10. Trained in the processes of sterilization and disinfection, inspection, and troubleshooting equipment, and assembly of instrument trays

_____ 11. Maintain a "dry" surgical site by operating suction devices and appropriate use of surgical sponge

_____ 12. Ensures patient chart, including results of diagnostic procedures, permits, and preoperative checklist accompany the patient in surgery

_____ 13. Prepares instruments and supplies on the sterile field

_____ 14. Nonsterile person who performs patient care procedures, obtains and delivers the equipment needed for a surgery case, opens sterile supplies, and assists in positioning the patient on the operating table

_____ 15. Maintains patient safety and follows emergency protocols as required

_____ 16. Assists surgeon in specific, well-defined tasks as needed during a procedure

a. Scrubbed surgical technologist

b. Circulator

c. Assistant circulator

d. Second assistant

e. Preceptor

f. Instrumentation specialist

g. Leadership and management

MULTIPLE CHOICE

1. The stated goals of a career ladder include all of the following, *except:*
   a. Improve patient care
   b. Promote accountability
   c. Encourage employer recognition of the surgical technologist
   d. Encourage experienced surgical technologists to contribute to the professional growth of their own career

2. The nonsterile member of the surgical team is called the:
   a. Technologist
   b. Scrub
   c. Circulator
   d. Surgeon

3. The surgical technologist who works in a hospital or other facility that provides 24-hour care is usually required to:
   a. Take a break every hour
   b. Take call
   c. work a 24-hour shift
   d. Work overtime

4. The role of the surgical technologist includes four main areas of health care and technology, *except:*
   a. Educator and preceptor
   b. Participant in leadership and management
   c. Patient care provider in the perioperative setting
   d. Specialist in sterilization

5. James is a new graduate, he is looking for a job in surgical technology, and career services has met with him and had him fill out applications for the following jobs:
   a. CST in general surgery
   b. Central processing manager
   c. Veterans Administration hospital, surgical technologist position
   d. CST on orthopedic team
   e. Medical equipment company representative
   f. Surgical Educator
   Of the above job fields, which two does James not qualify to do as a new graduate? _____

6. _____ is an individual with particular attributes (attitude and behavior), which reflect a high standard of accountability, ethics, honesty, and respect for people.
   a. Someone highly trained
   b. Someone who uses his or her skills
   c. A professional
   d. A surgical technologist

7. _____ means that patients, their families, and others in the care environment maintain a high level of confidence in the professionals that care for them.
   a. Discretion
   b. Tact
   c. Honesty
   d. Public trust

8. _____ means to be trustworthy, reliable, and responsible, not only on the job, but at all times, in all areas of one's life.
   a. Punctuality
   b. Personal integrity
   c. Respect for the law
   d. Discretion

9. A person who is _____ maintains professional demeanor even under stress.
   a. emotionally mature
   b. honest
   c. respects rules, regulations, and laws
   d. discrete

10. Health professionals, including surgical technologists, are often confronted with difficult situations requiring diplomacy and tact. This personal attribute is enhanced by _____.
    a. studying surgical procedures
    b. watching the surgeon
    c. having good role models in the work place and community
    d. being well-liked in the work place

11. Erosion of good aseptic technique can occur _____ (multiple answers possible).
    a. in a clinical environment in which technique is poor
    b. as a person becomes more knowledgeable
    c. with stress on the job
    d. with peer pressure

12. The surgical technologist can achieve career goals in a variety of settings. These include the following *except:* _____.
    a. A large medical center
    b. Military service
    c. Pharmaceutical research center
    d. Surgicenter

CASE STUDIES

1. Read the following case study and answer the questions based on your knowledge of the scope of practice for a surgical technologist:

You are a surgical technologist who has been hired as a new graduate in the local surgery center. You have worked there for about a month, and a seasoned certified surgical technologist is still acting as your preceptor. You have been assigned to work with Dr. Smith, who will be performing an open inguinal hernia procedure. You have never worked with this surgeon before. Once the procedure begins, the surgeon asks you to administer the local anesthetic. You know that as a surgical technologist, you are not allowed to administer medications.

a. Are you required to perform tasks delegated by the surgeon?

b. Is administration of a local anesthetic within your scope of practice?

c. Can you perform this delegated task if the surgeon states that he will take the responsibility?

d. What could you do in this situation?

2. *Read the following case study and answer the questions based on your knowledge of certification options for a surgical technologist:*

You have worked in an operating room for the past 15 years. Your hospital recently merged with another local hospital. The new combined hospital has asked that all surgical technologists become certified within the next 12 months. You were trained on the job; you did not graduate from an accredited program, and you are not eligible to take the examination through the NBSTSA.

a. Can you become certified?

b. What are your other options for certification?

c. What are the requirements for the alternate certification process?

d. If you were to become certified with one of the options you listed, do you have to take a national examination?

e. What would your title be if you became certified with the organization you listed in the first question?

f. If you are not certified with the NBSTSA, can you join the Association of Surgical Technologists?

2 Communication and Teamwork

Student's Name _____

KEY TERMS

Write the definition for each term.

1. Aggression: _____

2. Assertiveness: _____

3. Body language: _____

4. Consensus: _____

5. Emoticon: _____

6. Facilitator: _____

7. Feedback: _____

8. Groupthink: _____

9. Lateral abuse: _____

10. Message: _____

11. Norms: _____

12. Receiver: _____

13. Sender: _____

14. Sexual harassment: _____

15. Therapeutic touch: _____

16. Verbal abuse: _____

17. Win-lose solution: _____

18. Win-win solution: _____

SHORT ANSWERS

Provide a short answer for each question or statement.

1. The operating room environment is stressful and may require long hours, insufficient breaks, and sometimes verbal abuse, which can result in loss of morale and may lead to burnout. This downward spiral can be prevented. What have you learned about how to avoid burnout?

   _____

   _____

2. When we speak as we would like to be spoken to, we are:

   _____

   _____

3. Briefly explain the phrase "touch is almost never neutral."

   _____

   _____

4. Is touch a privilege earned by trust and limited by the boundaries of culture and social custom?

   _____

   _____

5. Does purposeful touch convey empathy, tenderness, and care?

   _____

   _____

6. Allowing others to think carefully before speaking shows _____ .

7. What are the elements of positive listening skills?

   _____

   _____

8. In the operating room, where communication often is rushed, the sender should look for _____, or body language, in the receiver to make sure the message has been received.

9. What environmental barriers to good communication are common in the operating room?

_____

_____

10. How is feedback given?

_____

_____

11. Many people begin to formulate a response before they have heard everything the sender has to say. Their thoughts are focused on what they want to say, and they fail to receive the message. What can you do to make sure you have been heard?

_____

_____

12. How does lateral abuse affect the work environment?

_____

_____

13. How can the receiver of verbal abuse approach the abuser?

_____

_____

14. How do you deal with problem behaviors in the operating room?

_____

_____

15. What is sexual harassment, and how does one deal with it in the operating room?

_____

_____

MATCHING

Match each term with the correct definition regarding communication. Some terms may be used more than once.

_____ 1. "I want to report that Dr. X broke another pair of scissors because they weren't sharp enough. Please speak with him."

_____ 2. "Dr. X's favorite elevators aren't on the ortho cart and they weren't with the other instruments. Would you mind calling upstairs? I need to scrub."

_____ 3. "Can you tell Dr. X that his 2 o'clock has been cancelled because the patient refused to sign the permit?" The patient's sitting in the holding room.

_____ 4. Focusing on the situation at hand, not allowing your thoughts to wander.

_____ 5. This used to ensure that the message was communicated correctly.

_____ 6. Requires active participation

_____ 7. Is nonjudgmental

_____ 8. Message is delivered without ambiguity or unnecessary information

a. Active listening

b. Assertiveness

c. Respect

d. Clarity

e. Feedback

MATCHING

Choose from the terms listed and match them with their most correct description. You may use an answer more than once.

_____ 1. One person may perceive an unemotional patient as a "stoic," and strong, brave person facing illness. Another person may see the same patient as extremely anxious and fearful, speechless, and unable to express emotion because of the intensity of his or her emotions.

_____ 2. How we perceive a problem, situation, or action sometimes depends on our social and cultural background as much as our knowledge.

_____ 3. Is an effective communication stopper

_____ 4. How we feel at the time of communication

_____ 5. Receiver does not have sufficient knowledge to understand exactly what the sender is trying to communicate

_____ 6. Hearing is a particular problem in the operating room

_____ 7. To be successful in sending and receiving information, a person must want to communicate

a. Emotions

b. Environmental barriers

c. Lack of a desire to communicate

d. Perceptions

e. Bias

f. Lack of understanding

g. Social and cultural influences

MULTIPLE CHOICE

Choose the most correct answer to complete the question or statement.

1. Communication should take place with the:
   a. Right person, time, and place
   b. Right time, person, and situation
   c. Right situation, person, and place
   d. Right person, place, and things

2. Who is the "right person" to communicate a problem with in the work place?
   a. Top management in all situations so that you are sure the message reaches the most authoritative person.
   b. Someone who seems to have the right answers most of the time
   c. One who can sympathize with the problem
   d. One who has the authority to help solve the problem

3. _____ maintains appropriate social boundaries when speaking to patients in the healthcare environment.
   a. A professional
   b. A department manager
   c. An instructor
   d. Someone who is mature in age

4. A professional's attire communicates a sense of responsibility and _____.
   a. Attitude
   b. Accountability
   c. Professionalism
   d. Awareness

5. The professional understands that most patients _____
   a. are afraid and worried
   b. do not understand the surgery or its risks
   c. have a high respect for health care workers
   d. are well informed about the surgery since they must sign the surgical consent

6. The operating room requires its personnel to work at a high level of mental, physical, and emotional strength. Because of this environment, the work is:
   a. Necessary
   b. Good
   c. Stressful
   d. Rehearsed

7. When team members have little knowledge of each other's work styles and personalities, then _____ is necessary.
   a. Close teamwork
   b. Verbal communication
   c. Personal space
   d. Organizational skills

8. The model for team relationships is _____.
   a. Respect for others
   b. A positive attitude
   c. Professionalism
   d. In transition

9. When working with people with problem behaviors, one must remember to focus on the behavior and not the _____.
   a. Person
   b. Attitude
   c. Team
   d. Task

10. Verbal abuse is a significant problem in the _____.
    a. Professional environment
    b. Operating room
    c. Family and work
    d. Work environment

11. What is verbal abuse:
    a. Vulgar remarks
    b. Violent public criticism demeaning another person
    c. Loud and abrasive comments or demands
    d. All the above

12. Verbal abuse sometimes is built into the operating room _____.
    a. Culture
    b. Environment
    c. Management
    d. Surgeons

13. Many people are reluctant to report abuse in the workplace for fear of:
    a. Retaliation
    b. Losing their job
    c. More abuse
    d. Administration

14. _____ abuse takes place among staff members of equal rank and position.
    a. Lateral
    b. Verbal
    c. Vertical
    d. Physical

15. Sexual harassment is an extreme abuse of power in which a person engages in the following types of behavior:
    a. Expects sexual favors in exchange for personal or professional gain
    b. Directs sexually explicit comments toward another
    c. Directs vulgar or sexual innuendoes at another
    d. All the above

16. Victims of sexual harassment should confront the perpetrator when sexual harassment occurs and afterward submit:
    a. A written report
    b. An oral report
    c. Nothing
    d. Documentation

17. A _____ is a group of people who come together to reach a common goal or set of goals.
    a. Gang
    b. Team
    c. Professional
    d. None of the above

18. Setting team priorities requires a _____
    a. Group
    b. Team
    c. Consensus
    d. A leader

19. Most role confusion is a result of poor:
    a. Teamwork
    b. Groupthink
    c. Attitude
    d. Communication

20. The goal of conflict resolution is to attempt to find a solution that is acceptable to all parties; this is called a _____-_____ solution.
    a. Win lose
    b. Win win
    c. Conflict resolution
    d. Open minded

21. A manager who makes most decisions with little or no input from the team is referred to as:
    a. Laissez-faire
    b. Democratic
    c. Experienced in groups
    d. Authoritarian

22. In the role of _____, the surgical technologist tutors the student and shares the duties of a scrubbed technologist.
    a. Team leader
    b. Preceptor
    c. Manager
    d. Instructor

CASE STUDIES

1. *You are a student who is about to graduate and is offered a job at your extern site. The surgeon you are working with is making sexual comments that make you feel uncomfortable.*

   a. What should you do?

   b. Why is documentation so important in issues involving sexual harassment?

c. Is this sexual harassment?

d. How do you know it is sexual harassment?

2. *Read the following scenario and then answer the questions that follow:*

You are in the operating room and scrubbed in for an exploratory laparotomy. The anesthesiologist and your circulator are chatting about a movie they both recently saw. The surgeon remains focused on the field. At this point there is increased hemorrhage and the surgery becomes more intense. You interrupt the circulator in her conversation to alert her to the sudden hemorrhage, and ask for more sponges.

After the patient has been taken to the postanesthesia care unit (PACU) and is stable, your circulator comes to you and states that you made her look "stupid" in front of the surgeon and the anesthesiologist.

a. Is the circulator's evaluation of the situation valid?

b. How do you respond to her?

c. What is the real issue here, and does it matter who is right?

3 Law, Documentation, and Professional Ethics

Student's Name _____

KEY TERMS

Write the definition for each term.

1. Abandonment: _____

2. Accountability: _____

3. Administrative Law: _____

4. Advance directive: _____

5. Damages: _____

6. Defamation: _____

7. Delegation: _____

8. Deposition: _____

9. Dilemma: _____

10. Ethical dilemma: _____

11. Ethics: _____

12. Evidenced based practice: _____

13. Hospital policy: _____

14. Incident report: _____

15. Informed consent: _____

16. Insurance: _____

17. Laws: _____

18. Liable: _____

19. Libel: _____

20. Living will: _____

21. Malpractice: _____

22. Medical ethics: _____

23. Medical power of attorney: _____

24. Negligence: _____

25. Perjury: _____

26. Practice acts: _____

27. Professional ethics: _____

28. Punitive: _____

29. Retained foreign object: _____

30. Safe Medical Devices Act: _____

31. Sentinel event: _____

32. Sexual harassment: _____

33. Slander: _____

34. Standard of conduct: _____

35. Statutes: _____

36. Subpoena: _____

37. TIMEOUT: _____

38. Tort: _____

39. Unretrieved device fragment: _____

SHORT ANSWERS

Provide a short answer for each question or statement.

1. Honoring the patient's privacy is a standard of conduct established by all health professions. This is a part of the code of conduct for hospitals. What are other standards of practice for surgical technologists?

   _____

   _____

Chapter **3** **Law, Documentation, and Professional Ethics**   Copyright © 2013, 2010, 2005 by Saunders, an imprint of Elsevier Inc.

2. What are the requirements for the delegation of a task?

_____

_____

3. What is accountability, and how does it apply to the surgical technologist's role in the healthcare facility?

_____

_____

4. What does the Latin phrase *respondeat superior* mean?

_____

_____

5. Who is responsible when a delegated task results in patient harm or injury?

_____

_____

6. In legal terms, what does it mean for a person to "do no harm"? Contrast that with what it means to the operating room team to "do no harm." Are they the same?

_____

_____

7. Can an approved hospital policy contradict the law of the state?

_____

_____

8. What is negligence?

_____

_____

9. What are the four elements of negligence that must be proven in a lawsuit?

_____

_____

10. Under what circumstances is it appropriate for a surgical technologist to refuse to take part in certain types of procedures?

_____

_____

11. Why is documentation so important? Explain the medical consequences of poor documentation.

_____

_____

MATCHING

Choose from the terms listed and match them with their most correct description. You may use the same answer more than once.

_____ 1. Decisions made by a court based on previous similar legal cases and decisions.

_____ 2. Standards that meet or exceed the Joint Commission

_____ 3. State laws

_____ 4. Violation may result in disciplinary action by the facility

_____ 5. Regulations passed by agencies and departments of the government such as the FDA

_____ 6. Practice acts

_____ 7. Logical, beneficial and created by specialists within the organization

_____ 8. Signed into law by its governor

_____ 9. Based on precedence from previous cases

_____ 10. Rules established by the Environmental Protection Agency (EPA) for the handling of medical waste

a. Hospital policy

b. Statutes

c. Administrative law

d. Legal doctrines

20

MULTIPLE CHOICE

Choose the correct answer for the question or statement.

1. You are scrubbed on a case in which the surgeons are discussing the patient's personal affairs which have no bearing on the surgical procedure or medical condition. These comments make you feel uncomfortable, you would consider this:
    a. Not your concern
    b. Lateral abuse
    c. Sexual harassment
    d. Slander

2. Tammy is a program director who frequently talks about her supervisor. Tammy informs the class that her supervisor is uneducated and does not know the standards and guidelines. These comments are:
    a. Defamation
    b. Negligent
    c. Assault
    d. Slander

3. _____ means deliberate efforts to erode the reputation of another person.
    a. Defamation
    b. Assault
    c. Battery
    d. Slander

4. _____ is the threat or attempt to harm another person.
    a. Battery
    b. False imprisonment
    c. Assault
    d. Slander

5. _____ involves contact with intent to injure and applies even if no injury occurred.
    a. Battery
    b. False imprisonment
    c. Assault
    d. Slander

6. Restraints become a method of managing a group of patients all in one place, possibly against their will. This type of case might be considered as:
    a. Battery
    b. False imprisonment
    c. Assault
    d. Slander

7. HIPAA protects a patient's _____ and other health information through its privacy rule.
    a. Medical Records
    b. Opinions
    c. Legal record including past convictions
    d. Constitutional rights

8. _____ represent a permanent legal record of the patient's interaction with health care providers and services.
    a. Laboratory results
    b. Surgical consent
    c. Documentation
    d. Forms

9. The _____ is the process in which the attending practitioner explains the risks, benefits, and alternatives of the surgery to the patient.
    a. Health literacy
    b. Signed consent
    c. Informed consent
    d. Discharge criteria

10. _____ _____ is the patient's ability to understand certain medical terminology used in the media and in educational settings.
    a. Informed consent
    b. HIPAA
    c. Health literacy
    d. Assessment benefits

11. The surgical consent is signed by the _____.
    a. Nurse and anesthesiologist
    b. Surgeon and family member
    c. Patient and anesthesiologist
    d. Patient and witness

12. A _____ is a legal document that specifically states the type of medical intervention or treatment the patient desires, in the event they are unable to speak for themselves in the future.
    a. Medical power of attorney
    b. Living will
    c. DNR
    d. None of the above

13. The surgical technologist has the right to abstain from participation in certain types of cases that violate his or her ethical, moral, or religious values. This is known as:
    a. Ethical dilemmas
    b. Refusal to perform an assigned task
    c. Moral dilemma
    d. All the above

1. *Read the following case study and answer the questions based on your knowledge of unintentional torts or civil wrongs.*

You have just been served with legal documents that suggest that you were scrubbed in on a procedure in which your patient was burned. You are charged with negligence. What reasons could you be charged for negligence in this situation?

2. *Read through the following case study. The areas of the scenario that are lettered and italicized are areas of potential negligence if the duties are not performed correctly. Write a brief sentence about each of the lettered and italicized areas to describe which area of civil or criminal liability applies:*

Your patient is being transported to the preanesthesia unit (PAU) by the transport team. The patient is accompanied by her neighbor, who will drive the patient home after the procedure.

When the team gets to the PAU, the room is empty. The transport team *(a) leaves the patient and (b) the chart* in the room to search for the nurse in charge. When the nurse gets to the room, she sedates the patient, as ordered on the chart by the anesthesiologist. The nurse notices that the patient has several necklaces on. She knows that the patient should not go into surgery wearing these, so she asks the patient to *(c) remove the necklaces*. She puts them loosely on the end of the patient's bed.

The nurse has been in the room for about 20 minutes and needs to check on the lab results. She asks a high school nurse's aide student *(d) to stand in the room* with the patient while she is gone. The aide is instructed to "holler for help" if she needs something.

When the nurse returns to the room, she notices that the consent form has not been signed. She *(e) asks the patient to sign the consent,* and (f) *asks the nurse's aide to witness.*

a. _____

b. _____

c. _____

d. _____

e. _____

f. _____

Chapter **3** **Law, Documentation, and Professional Ethics**

Student's Name _____

KEY TERMS

Write the definition for each term.

1. Accreditation: _____

2. Administration: _____

3. Air exchange: _____

4. Back table: _____

5. Biomedical engineering technician: _____

6. Case cart system: _____

7. Central core: _____

8. Chain of command: _____

9. Decontamination area: _____

10. Efficiency: _____

11. High-efficiency particulate air (HEPA) filters: _____

12. Integrated operating room: _____

13. Job description: _____

14. Job title: _____

15. Laminar airflow (LAF) system: _____

16. Organizational chart (Organigram): _____

17. Personnel policy: _____

18. Postanesthesia care unit (PACU): _____

19. Restricted area: _____

20. Risk management: _____

21. Role confusion: _____

22. Semirestricted area: _____

23. The Joint Commission: _____

24. Traffic patterns: _____

25. Transitional area: _____

26. Unrestricted area: _____

SHORT ANSWERS

Provide a short answer for each question or statement.

1. The surgical department is structured and engineered with three objectives in mind. List the three objectives.

    a. _____

    b. _____

    c. _____

2. Traffic patterns in the operating room are restricted. Describe the typical traffic pattern for an operating room, and explain why the movement is restricted.

    _____

    _____

3. Explain how airflow in the operating room is managed to prevent infection.

    _____

    _____

4. Explain the HEPA air filtering system.

    _____

    _____

5. Instruments that are particularly delicate (e.g., eye or those used in microsurgery) might not go to the sterile processing room. What is a more appropriate way to process instruments such as these after a surgical procedure?

    _____

    _____

6. The operating room could not function without the collaborative efforts of professionals outside the OR. What major functions do these departments implement?

_____

_____

7. Who is the operating room educator, and what are the job duties of this person in the operating room?

_____

_____

8. Explain how the chain of command and the organizational chart are interrelated.

_____

_____

9. Design an operating room suite to include all ancillary departments.

MATCHING

Match each term with the correct definition. Some terms may be used more than once.

_____ 1. High risk associated with electrosurgical devices

_____ 2. Oxygen, compressed air, nitrous oxide, and nitrogen are available through inline systems

_____ 3. Surgical doors must remain closed to maintain positive pressure differential

_____ 4. Derived from LED

_____ 5. Installed in the operating room ventilation system and removes particles

_____ 6. When the door is opened, positive pressure from within the room pushes air out and prevents it from entering the suite

_____ 7. 400 to 600 exchanges per hour

_____ 8. Must be maintained at 68 degrees to 73 degrees

_____ 9. Must be changed on a regular basis

_____ 10. Function is to move a large volume of air containing particles and microorganisms out of the operating room

_____ 11. Must be kept at 30% to 60%

_____ 12. Used as adjuncts to anesthesia and as a power source during surgical procedure

_____ 13. Numerous codes related to the types of outlets used

_____ 14. Energy is emitted by both halogen and LED

a. Airflow and ventilation

b. High-efficiency particulate air (HEPA) filter

c. Laminar airflow (LAF) system

d. Humidity and temperature

e. Lighting

f. Gases

g. Electricity

MATCHING

Choose from the terms listed and match them with their most correct description. You may use the same answer more than once.

_____ 1. Is constructed of stainless steel and fitted into a wheeled frame

_____ 2. Holds instruments and supplies except those for immediate use

_____ 3. Small tables used for skin prep kits, power equipment, and extra sterile supplies

_____ 4. Smaller table with one open end that can be raised and lowered

_____ 5. Is covered with a firm removable pad

_____ 6. Holds wrapped basin sets

_____ 7. Designated for soiled surgical sponges

_____ 8. Is covered with a sterile drape and used for instruments and supplies that are needed immediately during surgery

_____ 9. Sterile pack is placed and opened on this piece of equipment

_____ 10. Is designed to support the lip of the basin

a. Back table

b. Mayo stand

c. Ring stand

d. Kick bucket

e. Prep tables

f. Operating room table

MULTIPLE CHOICE

Choose the most correct answer to complete the question or statement.

1. _____ is the economic use of time and energy to save unnecessary work, material resources, and time.
   a. Efficiency
   b. Engineering
   c. Environment
   d. Operations

2. _____ are physical routes for people and equipment in the health care facility, which are designed to prevent the transmission of disease.
   a. Airflow
   b. Traffic patterns
   c. Clean area
   d. Certain areas

3. The department is separated into three distinct areas:
   a. Restricted, semirestricted, and clean
   b. Unrestricted, clean, and dirty
   c. Unrestricted, clean, and restricted
   d. Unrestricted, semirestricted, and restricted

4. People entering the operating room department proceed directly into the _____ area.
   a. Restricted
   b. Unrestricted
   c. Semirestricted
   d. None of the above

5. Only personnel in complete scrub attire, including hair cap, mask, and facial hair covering, are permitted in the _____ area.
   a. Restricted
   b. Unrestricted
   c. Semirestricted
   d. None of the above

6. The _____ core contains clean and sterile equipment and supplies.
   a. Clean
   b. Sterile
   c. Central
   d. Equipment

7. The primary design goal of the floor plan is to create a clear separation between _____ and _____ equipment.
   a. Sterile, clean
   b. Soiled, contaminated
   c. Soiled, clean
   d. Dirty, soiled

8. _____ in the surgical suite are stored in closed cabinets to keep them clean.
   a. Sterile supplies
   b. The computer and accessories
   c. Anesthesia drugs
   d. Anesthesia hoses and masks

9. The operating room table is adjustable for height, degree of tilt in all directions, orientation in the room, articular breaks, and _____.
   a. patient weight capacity
   b. ability to be used for transport
   c. safety features
   d. length

10. The back table is a large, stainless steel table on which all instruments, supplies, and equipment needed for surgery are arranged, except for those needed for:
    a. immediate use
    b. delivery of anesthesia
    c. later in the case
    d. suturing

CASE STUDIES

1. *Read the following case study and, using the information given, draw an organizational chart:*

You have just been hired at your local hospital. Mr. Hall is the chief administrator. He has also just been hired. He asks you if you could show him the chain of command for your area of surgical services. Because you work in a very small hospital, there are only two certified surgical technologists, you and one other scrub (Arlinda). Two nurses (Paul and Lydia) work in the OR. When you are scrubbed, you work mostly with Dr. May and Dr. Smith.

The charge nurse for your area is Mrs. Jones. She has worked at the hospital in this position for 25 years. The operating room staff educator's name is Abby. Mrs. Markus is the operating room nurse manager, and she reports to the director of perioperative services. His name is Mr. Smith. Mr. Smith reports to the vice president of patient care services, Mr. Zander.

a. Design an organization chart, and define each role in the chart.

b. Design a chain of command in surgery.

2. *You have just been hired as a new surgical technologist. You are opening supplies for your case and you notice that the circulator and extra scrub tech are not opening the supplies correctly.*

As you watch, you see several breaks in techniques, as a new employee:

a. Do you say anything?

b. What do you say?

c. Define surgical conscience. Does it apply here?

d. Who do you tell, and how do you approach them?

e. What effects will this have on the patient?

3. *Your hospital has been bought out. They are looking for a new design for the operating room and you have been chosen to be on the design team. They ask you to do the following:*

a. Design an operating room

b. Include all ancillary departments

c. Include any other items you feel will enhance the department

5 Disaster Preparedness and Response

Student's Name _____

KEY TERMS

Write the definition for each term.

1. Agency for Healthcare Research and Quality (AHRQ): _____

2. All-hazards approach: _____

3. American Red Cross: _____

4. Bioterrorism: _____

5. Declared state of emergency: _____

6. Disaster: _____

7. Disaster recovery: _____

8. Emergency: _____

9. Federal Emergency Management Agency (FEMA): _____

10. Logistics supply chain: _____

11. Mass casualty event: _____

12. Medical Reserve Corps: _____

13. Mitigation: _____

14. National Disaster Life Support Education Consortium (NDLSEC): _____

15. National Disaster Medical System (NDMS): _____

16. National Fire Protection Agency (NFPA): _____

17. Natural disaster: _____

18. Pandemic: _____

19. Shelter-in-place: _____

20. Surge capacity: _____

21. Vulnerability: _____

SHORT ANSWERS

Provide a short answer for each question or statement.

1. What is the difference between a disaster and an emergency?

   _____

   _____

2. List types of weather-related disasters.

   _____

   _____

3. List types of human made disasters.

   _____

   _____

4. What is bioterrorism?

   _____

   _____

5. Define the three levels of disasters.

   _____

   _____

6. What role does the community play in disaster preparation?

   _____

   _____

7. List the primary objectives of a local disaster plan.

   _____

   _____

MATCHING

Match each term with the correct definition.

_____ 1. An important activity in infection control during a disaster

_____ 2. Ensures that a disaster response is consistent with the doctrines and laws of the country

_____ 3. A process in which people are physically moved away from the environmental dangers caused by a disaster

_____ 4. A process of bringing family members in contact during and after a disaster

_____ 5. Social and psychological assistance needed in every disaster

_____ 6. Protects people from harsh environmental conditions

_____ 7. Form the process of transport and distribution of materials, goods, food, and other necessary supplies

_____ 8. A designated area for placing the dead which is removed from public areas

a. Shelter

b. Evacuation

c. Temporary Morgue

d. Logistics

e. Mental health needs

f. Health messages in the community

g. Department of Homeland Security

h. Reunification

MULTIPLE CHOICE

Choose the most correct answer for each question or statement.

1. _____ is a process in which casualties are given emergency medical treatment according to the probability of their survival.
   a. Surge capacity
   b. Communication
   c. Triage
   d. Medical facility evacuation

2. A major health facility has the ability to _____ using satellite or high frequency radio.
   a. analyze surge capacity
   b. communicate
   c. perform Triage
   d. evacuate injured people

3. _____ of a medical facility may sometimes be necessary because of structural hazards or immediate threat from fire, chemical, or bioterrorism.
   a. Surge capacity
   b. Communication
   c. Triage
   d. Evacuation

4. _____ is the ability of a health care facility to quickly increase its capability to receive and treat patients.
   a. Surge capacity
   b. Communication
   c. Triage
   d. Medical facility evacuation

5. Roles are assigned using a *job action sheet* (JAS). This is a tool used to define
   a. Surge capacity
   b. Staff assignments
   c. Triage
   d. Medical facility management team

6. During a disaster, individual health care workers may be asked to:
   a. perform tasks outside their scope of practice
   b. perform tasks outside their usual role.
   c. perform management tasks even though they have no experience
   d. be a spokesperson for the hospital

7. During a disaster, the press and other media require:
   a. food and water from the health facility
   b. the ability to examine patients
   c. lists of the dead
   d. a designated communication area to be based

1. *Read the following case study and answer the questions based on your knowledge of the health care disaster plan:*

   You are a CST and you are at home when a tornado hits your community:

   a. What is your first response?

   b. After you secure your family, what should you do next?

2. *Read the following case study and answer the questions based on your knowledge of the ethical dilemmas in a disaster:*

   You are a CST working during a hurricane. You have worked over 12 hours with no breaks for dinner. Your coworkers cannot get to the hospital due to the disaster. Answer the following questions:

   a. Should you refuse to work any longer?

b. What do you do if your husband has to have immediate surgery and there is no one there to relieve you?

c. What are your ethical responsibilities during a disaster.

6 The Patient

Student's Name _____

KEY TERMS

Write the definition for each term.

1. Body image: _____

2. Cultural competence: _____

3. Elimination: _____

4. Maslow's hierarchy of human needs: _____

5. Mobility: _____

6. Nutrition: _____

7. Patient-centered care: _____

8. Physiological: _____

9. Reflection: _____

10. Therapeutic communication: _____

SHORT ANSWERS

Provide a short answer for each question or statement.

1. What is the patient-centered care?

   _____

   _____

2. What does Maslow's chart teach us about the needs of individuals?

   _____

   _____

3. Why would a patient feel a loss of security if he or she were about to undergo a surgical procedure?

_____

_____

4. Why is self-image important to a patient before surgery?

_____

_____

5. Therapeutic communication includes:

_____

_____

6. List the specific risks of injury for the obese patient before, during, and after surgery.

_____

_____

7. Explain two different types of diabetes and how they can affect the outcome of the surgical patient.

_____

_____

8. Explain the golden hour.

_____

_____

9. Explain developmental disability and how it affects communication.

_____

_____

10. List some strategies for communicating with patients who understand limited English.

_____

_____

MATCHING

Define Maslow's triangular hierarchy with the correct definition and give an example of each.

1. _____ Sleep
2. _____ Temperature
3. _____ Mobility
4. _____ Safety
5. _____ Security
6. _____ Belonging
7. _____ Altered body image
8. _____ Achieving personal goals
9. _____ Elimination
10. _____ Respiration
11. _____ Love
12. _____ Nutrition

a. physiological
b. protection
c. relational
d. self-actualization

MULTIPLE CHOICE

Choose the most correct answer for each question or statement.

1. According to Maslow's hierarchy of needs, the most basic of human needs are _____.
   a. Psychological
   b. Physiological
   c. Metabolic
   d. Pathological

2. Maslow's hierarchy of human needs is depicted as a triangular hierarchy in which the critical needs to preserve life are at the base levels, and other needs that create the rest of the hierarchy are:
   a. Emotional
   b. Social
   c. Spiritual fulfillment
   d. All the above

3. A patient's fear that he or she will not awaken from the anesthetic, or will feel pain while remaining paralyzed is called:
   a. Anesthesia
   b. Anesthesia awareness
   c. Anesthesia provider
   d. Anesthetic agents

4. Fear of _____ during or after surgery is common among patients.
   a. Pain
   b. Disfigurement
   c. Loss of control
   d. Death

5. Fear of _____ is a normal protective mechanism.
   a. Pain
   b. Disfigurement
   c. Loss of control
   d. Death

6. Patients undergoing radical or reconstructive surgery have realistic fears about:
   a. Pain
   b. Disfigurement
   c. Loss of control
   d. Death

7. When patients enter the health care system, they often feel a loss of personal rights and _____.
   a. Pain
   b. Disfigurement
   c. Control
   d. Death

8. The fear of _____ of the body is quite strong in many patients, especially adolescents.
   a. Pain exposure
   b. Physical exposure
   c. Control
   d. Death

9. _____ are powerful needs.
   a. Acceptance and nurturing
   b. Support and family
   c. Love and belonging
   d. All the above

10. Many patients are afraid that information about their health may not be held in confidence. This is a fear of:
    a. Loss of privacy
    b. Physical exposure
    c. Control
    d. Death

11. _____ of acceptance, or being accepted, contribute to a healthy ego and the ability to pursue goals and objectives in life.
    a. Emotions
    b. Needs
    c. Control
    d. Feelings

12. Maslow's model includes _____ and self-image because the perception we have of ourselves influences motivation and relationships, both social and personal.
    a. Self-esteem
    b. Feelings of acceptance
    c. Family needs
    d. Self-doubt

13. _____ is not only dependent on physical appearance but also on people's normal roles within their family and community.
    a. Self-esteem
    b. Feelings of acceptance
    c. Family needs
    d. Self-image

CASE STUDIES

1. *Read the following case study and answer the questions based on your knowledge of therapeutic communication and geriatric patients:*

You have been asked by the operating room (OR) supervisor to help transport an elderly patient to the preop holding area from her patient room. The patient was recently diagnosed with breast cancer. You enter the patient's room and introduce yourself. The following conversation ensues:

You: "Hello, sweetie. My name is Jane Smith, and I'm here to transport you to surgery today. Can you please tell me the name of your surgeon and the type of procedure you will be having today?"

Mrs. Smith: "Dr. Woods is my surgeon, and he is going to remove my cancer today."

You: "Could you be more specific, Mrs. Smith? Where is your cancer?"

Mrs. Smith: "The cancer is in my left breast. (pause) I'm worried about the surgery. My friend said that the procedure is very disfiguring."

You: "Many patients are afraid of surgery, Mrs. Smith."

Mrs. Smith: "I'm worried that I might die from the cancer if the doctor doesn't get it all out."

You: "Would you like to talk to someone about this before we go to surgery?"

Mrs. Smith: "No, I guess not. I'm ready to go."

You: "Okay, can I get you to scoot over to the OR stretcher for me?"

Now answer the following questions about this conversation:

a. Are you comfortable with the way this conversation has gone?

b. Was the conversation helpful in alleviating the patient's fear before you brought her to surgery?

c. Is the conversation you are having with the patient helpful or therapeutic?

d. Modify the conversation so that it becomes therapeutic for the patient. Change your responses above.

2. *Read the following case study and answer the questions based on your knowledge of patient rights and cultural competency.*

You are a CST and your job today in the OR is to assist the circulator with her duties. Your patient arrives in the operating room. He has prayer beads and a religious item that you do not recognize from your own religious practice. You do not know anything about his religion. You are assisting the procedure for a general anesthetic and placing the patient monitors on your patient. He states that he is "afraid" and asks you to pray with him before he goes to sleep.

Answer the following questions about this patient's care.

a. What can you do now to ease his fear?

b. Can he keep his religious items with him during the procedure?

c. How can you pray with him and still retain your own religious and spiritual beliefs and his as well?

d. Evaluate the statement, "Caregivers do not have to have cancer to understand the process" with regard to this patient.

3. *In a group, design a Maslow's hierarchy needs chart.*

    a. Give an example of each area and how it pertains to the surgical patient.

    b. How does the hierarchy relate to the CST during care of the surgical patient.

    c. What happens if one area is not given the right attention at the right time?

7 Diagnostic and Assessment Procedures

Student's Name _____

KEY TERMS

Write the definition for each term.

1. ABO blood group _____

2. Acute illness _____

3. Benign _____

4. Chronic illness _____

5. Complete blood count (CBC) _____

6. Computed tomography (CT) _____

7. Contrast medium _____

8. Diastolic pressure _____

9. Differential count _____

10. Doppler studies _____

11. Electrocardiography _____

12. Endoscopic procedures _____

13. Fluoroscopy _____

14. Hematocrit (Hct) _____

15. Hemoglobin (Hgb) _____

16. Imaging studies _____

17. Invasive procedure _____

18. Magnetic resonance imaging _____

19. Malignant _____

20. Mean arterial pressure (MAP) _____

21. Metastasis _____

22. Neoplasm _____

23. Nuclear medicine _____

24. Orthostatic (postural) blood pressure _____

25. Palpating _____

26. Partial thromboplastin time (PTT) _____

27. Positron emission tomography (PET) _____

28. Prothrombin time _____

29. Pulse pressure _____

30. Radioactive seed _____

31. Radionuclide or isotopes _____

32. Radiopaque _____

33. Sphygmomanometer _____

34. Staging _____

35. Systolic pressure _____

36. TNM classification system _____

37. Transcutaneous _____

38. Tumor marker _____

39. Vital signs _____

SHORT ANSWERS

Provide a short answer for each question or statement.

1. The vital signs include:

   _____

   _____

2. During surgery, why is it important to monitor vital signs?

   _____

   _____

3. What is the difference between acute and chronic illness?

   a. Give an example of each.

     _____

     _____

4. What are the five different ways a patient's temperature might be taken?

   a. _____

   b. _____

   c. _____

   d. _____

   e. _____

5. Explain the three- or four-point scale used to report the strength of the pulse, as well as the terminology used to describe the pulse.

     _____

     _____

     _____

     _____

     _____

6. Describe the technique for measuring the respiratory rate.

     _____

     _____

7. Describe the technique of evaluating the pulse using the associated terms and definitions.

     _____

     _____

     _____

8. List the areas for measuring the pulse.

     _____

     _____

9. What can alter the respiratory rate?

_____

_____

10. What problems are associated with evaluation of a patient's blood pressure using a simple digital (automatic) sphygmomanometer?

_____

_____

_____

11. Pressure varies by age and is affected by various other normal physiological conditions, including:

_____

_____

12. Important normal physiological factors that influence blood pressure include:

_____

_____

13. List the technique for taking the blood pressure.

_____

_____

14. List the common errors associated with blood pressure measurement.

_____

_____

15. The CBC is a basic test used to evaluate the type and percentage of normal components in the blood. What five components are tested?

_____

_____

_____

_____

_____

16. Positively charged electrolytes are called *cations*. Which cations are routinely tested during a routine blood workup?

_____

_____

MATCHING

Match each term with the correct definition.

1. _____ Combines radiography with an image intensifier that is visible in normal lighting

2. _____ Is generated by high-frequency sound waves

3. _____ Uses radiofrequency signals and multiple magnetic fields to produce a high definition image

4. _____ Uses the combined technologies of computed tomography and radioactive scanning.

5. _____ X-ray and computer technologies are combined to produce high contrast cross-sectional images

a. Computed tomography (CT)

b. Magnetic resource imaging (MRI)

c. Fluoroscopy

d. Positron emission tomography (PET)

e. Ultrasound

MATCHING

1. _____ A person's blood type

2. _____ Is a basic test used to evaluate the type and percentage of normal components in the blood

3. _____ The mechanism of blood clotting

4. _____ Cations and anions

5. _____ Includes blood glucose, carbon dioxide, creatinine, urea nitrogen, bicarbonate, and several important electrolytes

6. _____ A measurement of these ions (bicarbonate and carbonic acid and provides a snapshot of this balancing mechanism.)

a. Complete blood count

b. Metabolic panel

c. Coagulation test

d. Arterial blood gases

e. ABO groups

f. Electrolytes

MULTIPLE CHOICE

Choose the most correct answer to complete the question or statement.

1. The most basic form of assessment.
   a. CT scan
   b. Chest radiograph
   c. ECG
   d. Vital signs

2. The body requires a core (deep) temperature of approximately 99° F, or
   a. 37.2° C
   b. 38.2° C
   c. 40° C
   d. 42° C

3. Axillary temperature readings are _____ than oral measurements.
   a. 0.3° to 0.6° C higher
   b. 0.5° to 1° F lower
   c. 0.5° C and 1.5° C lower
   d. 0.6° C and 1.6° C higher

4. Which statement about the use of thermometers is true?
   a. The use of external thermometers, such as the tympanic thermometer, poses less risk of infection for your patient.
   b. You do not need to wash your hands after taking a patient's temperature with a forehead or skin thermometer because it is not an invasive procedure.
   c. The rectal method is preferred over the tympanic method.
   d. Tympanic thermometers can harbor an infectious biofilm that may not be visible.

5. The normal pulse rate for an adult is _____.
   a. 40 to 60 beats per minute
   b. 60 to 100 beats per minute
   c. 75 to 110 beats per minute
   d. 80 to 120 beats per minute

6. The pulse range for an athlete is:
   a. 50 to 100 beats per minute
   b. 60 to 100 beats per minute
   c. 75 to 110 beats per minute
   d. 80 to 120 beats per minute

7. _____ provides detailed information about heart conduction.
   a. ECG
   b. EEG
   c. Blood pressure
   d. Oximetry

8. The basic metabolic panel includes all of the following, *except:*
   a. Blood glucose
   b. Carbon dioxide
   c. Creatinine
   d. Oxygen

9. _____ is performed to assess the functional ability of the coagulation sequence.
   a. Electrolyte testing
   b. ABO group testing
   c. PTT
   d. Measurement of ABG levels

10. Electrolytes include all the following, *except:*
    a. Sodium
    b. Carbonic acid
    c. Potassium
    d. Calcium

11. Hypocalcemia is caused from a deficiency of what electrolyte?
    a. Calcium
    b. Potassium
    c. Sodium
    d. None of the above

12. Hyponatremia is caused from a deficiency of what electrolyte?
    a. Calcium
    b. Potassium
    c. Sodium
    d. None of the above

13. Hypokalemia is caused from a deficiency of what electrolyte?
    a. Calcium
    b. Potassium
    c. Sodium
    d. None of the above

14. Urinalysis is performed to assess the body's overall health, with particular focus on the urinary tract; a simple screening is performed to check for different substances to include all, *except:*
    a. Albumin
    b. Glucose
    c. Magnesium
    d. Leukocytes

15. One of the tests used to detect infection is the
    a. Biopsy and aspiration
    b. Sensitivity and aspiration
    c. Culture and biopsy
    d. Culture and sensitivity

16. The surgical removal of a small portion of tissue is a(n)
    a. Needle or trocar biopsy
    b. Brush biopsy
    c. Excision
    d. Smear

17. Obtained by passing a swab or small brush over superficial tissue.
    a. Needle or trocar biopsy
    b. Brush biopsy
    c. Excision
    d. Smear

18. Used to sweep a hollow lumen or cavity for cells.
    a. Needle or trocar biopsy
    b. Brush biopsy
    c. Excision
    d. Smear

19. A core sample of tissue is removed in one or more locations of the suspected area.
    a. Needle or trocar biopsy
    b. Brush biopsy
    c. Excision
    d. Smear

20. Fluid for pathological examination may be removed using.
    a. Needle or trocar biopsy
    b. Brush biopsy
    c. Aspiration needle
    d. Smear

21. Tissue is removed and immediately placed in liquid nitrogen.
    a. Frozen section
    b. Brush biopsy
    c. Excision
    d. Smear

22. Abnormal growth
    a. Malignant tumor
    b. Benign tumor
    c. Metastasis
    d. Neoplasm

23. Is composed of cells belonging to a single tissue type and does not spread to distant regions of the body.
    a. Malignant tumor
    b. Benign tumor
    c. Metastasis
    d. Neoplasm

24. New tumors may develop from these "seed" cells.
    a. Malignant tumor
    b. Benign tumor
    c. Metastasis

25. Composed of disorganized tissue that exhibits uncontrolled growth.
    a. Malignant tumor
    b. Benign tumor
    c. Metastasis
    d. Neoplasm

CASE STUDIES

1. *Read the following case study and answer the questions based on your knowledge of temperature conversion. You are asked to take the patient's vital signs. You can only find one blood pressure cuff. It is intended for normal adults. Your patient's BMI is 40 (morbidly obese).*

   a. How will this cuff affect the blood pressure reading?

53

b. Can you use this cuff as long as you document which size you used?

c. While inflating the cuff, it suddenly pops off the patient's arm. How should you proceed?

8 Environmental Hazards

Student's Name _____

Write the definition for each term.

1. Airborne transmission precautions: _____

2. Blood-borne pathogens: _____

3. Electrocution: _____

4. Electrosurgical unit: _____

5. Eschar: _____

6. Flammable: _____

7. Grounding: _____

8. Hypersensitivity: _____

9. Impedance (resistance): _____

10. Latex: _____

11. Neutral zone (no hands) technique: _____

12. Occupational exposure: _____

13. Oxiders: _____

14. Oxygen-enriched atmosphere (OEA): _____

15. Personal protective equipment: _____

16. Postexposure prophylaxis: _____

17. Risk: _____

18. Sharps: _____

19. Smoke plume: _____

20. Standard Precautions: _____

21. Transmission-based precautions: _____

22. Underwriters Laboratories: _____

23. Volatile: _____

SHORT ANSWERS

Provide a short answer for each question or statement.

1. What are some common causes of occupational injury?

   _____

   _____

2. What is the fire triangle? How do the components relate to each other?

   _____

   _____

3. What is "source of ignition"?

   _____

   _____

4. What is a patient fire?

   _____

   _____

5. List several fuels that are capable of causing surgical site fires and explain how to prevent them.

   _____

   _____

6. Name the common sources of ignition found in the operating room.

   _____

   _____

7. What percentage of patient fires occurs inside or on the skin surface?

   _____

   _____

8. If a fire breaks out in the operating room, what three steps should be taken immediately to protect the patient and put out the fire?

_____

_____

9. What parts of a compressed gas cylinder should you inspect for safe operation?

_____

_____

10. Describe the recommended procedure for transporting compressed gas cylinders in the health care facility.

_____

_____

11. List the guidelines for storage of gas cylinders.

_____

_____

12. What is the leading cause of hospital fires in the United States?

_____

_____

13. What is a Material Safety Data Sheet?

_____

_____

14. Why are Standard Precautions used in healthcare?

_____

_____

15. What is the neutral zone (no hands) technique?

_____

_____

16. What is PEP, and what does it involve?

_____

_____

17. What diseases require airborne transmission precautions? Droplet precautions?

_____

_____

18. Name five methods that can be used to reduce the risk of sharps injuries.

_____

_____

19. How does clutter in the operating room contribute to skeletal injury?

_____

_____

20. What is the most common means of transmission of blood borne diseases in the health care setting?

_____

_____

Using the following triangle, draw in the three components required for fire. Under each of the three components, make a directory of the items specific to the operating room that fall into that section.

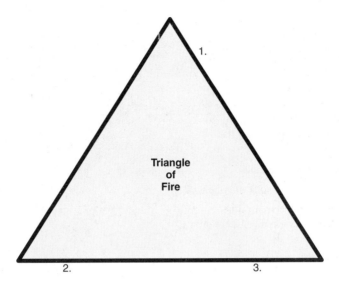

1. _____

_____

_____

2. _____

_____

_____

3. _____

_____

_____

MATCHING

Determine whether each statement refers to ionizing radiation (a) or magnetic resonance imaging (b).

1. _____ A lead apron must be worn during fluoroscopy to prevent exposure to scatter radiation.

2. _____ Lead aprons must be stored flat or hung in a manner that prevents bending of the material.

3. _____ Remember that a lead apron protects only the areas of the body that are covered by the apron.

4. _____ The primary risk is the presence of metal, which can be drawn from its source and into the path of the powerful magnetic field. For this reason, absolutely no metal objects are permitted in the environment during this process.

5. _____ The eyes and hands are not protected.

6. _____ Metal implants in the patient or staff members.

7. _____ Those who must remain in the room during exposure must maintain a distance of at least 6 feet (1.8 m) from the patient.

8. _____ Neck shields are available to protect the thyroid, which is sensitive to radiation, during fluoroscopy.

9. _____ Personal items, such as scissors or jewelry.

10. _____ Nonsterile workers should step outside the range of exposure, either behind a lead screen or outside the room.

11. _____ Only plastic and titanium objects are safe.

12. _____ Lead glasses should be worn during exposure to a fluoroscope.

13. _____ The safest place to stand is at a right angle to the beam on the side of the radiograph machine or origin of the radiation beam.

a. Ionizing radiation

b. Magnetic resonance imaging

MULTIPLE CHOICE

Choose the most correct answer to complete the question or statement.

1. Materials and substances that burn are called _____.
   a. Flammable
   b. Flame resistant
   c. Flame retardant
   d. High alert

2. Which of the following statements is true regarding the high fire risk in the operating room?
   a. Oxygen is heavier than air and settles on the floor.
   b. Oxygen is lighter than air and tends to float above the anesthesia machine.
   c. Oxygen may become confined in areas such as the groin and the axilla.
   d. When nitrous oxide decomposes in the presence of heat, oxygen molecules are produced, creating an oxygen-rich environment.

3. An environment that has a concentration of oxygen greater than 21% is called an _____ .
   a. Oxygen-poor atmosphere
   b. Oxygen-enriched atmosphere
   c. Operating room oxygen
   d. Oxidizer

4. Which of the following are considered flammable?
   a. Endotracheal tubes
   b. Surgical drapes
   c. Fibrin glue
   d. All of the above

5. Which of the following are considered sources of ignition?
   a. Surgical drapes
   b. Laser
   c. Chlorhexidine
   d. Alcohol Prepping solution

6. During a colonoscopy, the potential for fire is high because of the high concentration of _____.
   a. Flammable drapes and equipment
   b. Oxygen
   c. Laser emissions
   d. Methane gas

7. On which of the following would you use a class A fire extinguisher?
   a. Electrical fires
   b. Laser fires
   c. Flammable liquids
   d. Wood, paper, and cloth

8. Class B fire extinguishers are also called _____ extinguishers.
   a. Bromochlorodifluoromethane
   b. Carbon dioxide
   c. Hydrogen peroxide
   d. Water

9. Which of the following acronyms should you remember if you are trying to put out a fire?
   a. PASS
   b. RACE
   c. RICE
   d. PAST

10. Compressed _____ is used as a power source for instruments, such as drills, saws, and other high-speed tools.
    a. Oxygen
    b. Argon
    c. Nitrogen
    d. Nitrous oxide

11. Which of the following compressed medical gases is used as an anesthetic gas?
    a. Oxygen
    b. Nitrous oxide
    c. Argon
    d. Carbon dioxide

12. Chemicals that are transferred from larger containers to smaller containers must be labeled with the exact information found on the _____.
    a. MSDS sheets
    b. Original container
    c. OSHA regulation sheets
    d. Manufacturer's directions

13. _____ is/are known to contain benzene, hydrogen cyanide, formaldehyde, blood fragments, and viruses.
    a. Peracetic acid
    b. Formaldehyde
    c. Smoke plumes
    d. Filters

14. With regard to toxic chemicals in the operating room, which of the following statements is true?
    a. The cumulative effects can be much greater than the effects of any single exposure.
    b. Many of the chemicals are hazardous, but they usually produce only short-term effects.
    c. Guidelines for handling chemicals are designed to help in the development of risk strategies.
    d. Only the emergency department is required to maintain MSDS for chemicals.

15. Nonresistant materials include _____ .
    a. Metal
    b. Water
    c. Human body
    d. All of the above
    e. None of the above

16. The risk reduction strategy that is used after exposure to blood or other body fluids is called _____.
    a. PPE
    b. PEP
    c. PPP
    d. All the above

17. Measles is a type of _____ transmission.
    a. Droplet
    b. Airborne
    c. Contact
    d. Standard

18. Rubella is a type of _____ transmission.
    a. Droplet
    b. Airborne
    c. Contact
    d. Standard

19. Impetigo is a type of _____ transmission.
    a. Droplet
    b. Airborne
    c. Contact
    d. Standard

Chapter **8** **Environmental Hazards**

20. The Environmental Protection Agency (EPA) defines medical waste as any solid waste generated in the diagnosis, treatment, or immunization of humans or animals. The following are examples of medical waste, *except:*
    a. Culture dishes and other glassware
    b. Needles used to administer medications or draw blood
    c. Smoke plume
    d. Used stainless steel instruments

21. _____ is a naturally occurring sap obtained from rubber trees.
    a. OPA
    b. Radiation
    c. Latex
    d. None of the above

22. Scaling, drying, and cracks in skin are symptoms of what type of allergic skin reaction?
    a. Contact dermatitis (nonallergic)
    b. Allergic contact dermatitis
    c. Natural rubber latex allergy
    d. Hypersensitivity

23. _____ causes dermatitis on contact with the object.
    a. Contact dermatitis (nonallergic)
    b. Allergic contact dermatitis
    c. Natural rubber latex allergy
    d. Hypersensitivity

24. _____ is the amount of physical effort needed to perform a task, such as moving an object.
    a. Posture
    b. Repetitive motion
    c. Exertion
    d. Contact stress

25. _____ is excessive direct pressure against a sharp edge or hard surface.
    a. Posture
    b. Repetitive motion
    c. Exertion
    d. Contact stress

26. _____ is a critical component of musculoskeletal stress.
    a. Posture
    b. Repetitive motion
    c. Exertion
    d. Contact stress

27. _____ places stress on tendons and muscles.
    a. Posture
    b. Repetitive motion
    c. Exertion
    d. Contact stress

28. When _____, keep the object close to your body.
    a. Lifting
    b. Pushing and pulling
    c. Bending
    d. Standing

29. When _____, place one foot behind the other, back foot should be braced comfortably.
    a. Lifting
    b. Pushing and pulling
    c. Bending
    d. Standing

CASE STUDIES

1. *Read the following case study and answer the questions based on your knowledge of fire in the operating room:*

   You are scrubbed in with an endoscopic procedure. The surgeon has disconnected the light cord from the endoscope and placed it on the surgical drapes without turning it off.

   a. What can you say to the surgeon about safety related to this?

   b. What is your own role here?

2. *Read the following case study and answer the questions based on your knowledge of fire in the operating room:*

   You are searching the OR suite for something that smells as if it is overheating. You see that a C-arm fluoroscopy machine is plugged into the wall. While you are calling the radiology department to come and check out the machine, it bursts into flames.

   a. Using the acronym RACE, describe the actions you will take.

   R _____

   A _____

   C _____

   E _____

9 Microbes and the Process of Infection

Student's Name _____

KEY TERMS

Write the definition for each term.

1. Aerobes: _____

2. Aerosol droplets: _____

3. Anaerobes: _____

4. Bioburden: _____

5. Contaminated: _____

6. Cross-contamination: _____

7. Culture: _____

8. Diffusion: _____

9. Direct transmission: _____

10. Droplet nuclei: _____

11. Endospore: _____

12. Entry site: _____

13. Fomite: _____

14. Infection: _____

15. Inflammation: _____

16. Necrosis: _____

17. Nosocomial infection: _____

18. Opportunistic infection: _____

19. Pathogen: _____

20. Prion: _____

21. Resident microorganism: _____

22. Sterile: _____

23. Suppurative: _____

24. Vector: _____

25. Virion: _____

26. Virulence: _____

LABELING

Label the following drawing of a prokaryotic cell. Make sure to use medical terminology where appropriate.

1. _____

2. _____

3. _____

4. _____

5. _____

prokaryote

From Goering R, Dockrell H, Wakelin D, et al: *Mim's medical microbiology*, ed 4, St Louis, 2008, Mosby.

Label the following drawing of a eukaryotic cell. Make sure to use medical terminology where appropriate.

1. _____

2. _____

3. _____

4. _____

5. _____

6. _____

7. _____

8. _____

eukaryote

From Goering R, Dockrell H, Wakelin D, et al: *Mim's medical microbiology*, ed 4, St Louis, 2008, Mosby.

SHORT ANSWERS

Provide a short answer for each question or statement.

1. Why is it important to identify microbes in the disease process?

   _____

   _____

2. What is a bacterial culture? Why do we perform this procedure?

   _____

   _____

3. How does the number of disease microbes at the site of entry relate to the process of infection?

   _____

   _____

4. List the tools for identifying microbes and give an example of each.

   _____

   _____

5. A surgical site infection may start as an abscess. What exactly is an abscess?

   _____

   _____

6. Why are bacteria the focus of study in disease microbiology?

   _____

   _____

7. List the most important methods of disease prevention in the health care facility.

   _____

   _____

MATCHING

Match the microbe with the correct definition and example.

1. _____ an organism lives on or within another organism (the host) and gains an advantage at the expense of that organism.

2. _____ one organism uses another to meet its physiological needs but causes no harm to the host. For example, the normal human intestinal tract contains many different types of bacteria, such as *Escherichia coli,* that are essential for metabolism.

3. _____ only about 3% to 5% of all microbes are pathogenic. However, nonpathogenic microbes (those that do not usually cause disease) that live in and on the body can become pathogenic under certain conditions.

4. _____ each of the organisms benefits from their relationship in the environment. For example, *Staphylococcus aureus* inhabits normal, healthy skin.

a. Commensalism

b. Mutualism

c. Parasitism

d. Opportunistic organisms

MATCHING

Match the disease transmission with the proper term.

1. _____ Staphylococcus aureus

2. _____ Talking, coughing, or sneezing

3. _____ Food

4. _____ Blood-borne pathogens

5. _____ Vector

a. Direct contact

b. Airborne transmission

c. Transmission by body fluids

d. Oral transmission (ingestion)

e. Fly

MULTIPLE CHOICE

Choose the most correct answer to complete the question or statement.

1. Virology is the study of _____.
   a. Disease mechanisms, diagnosis, and treatment
   b. Bacteria
   c. Microbes
   d. Viruses

2. Which of the following is *not* a characteristic of eukaryotic cells?
   a. Multicellular
   b. Double-layer membrane
   c. Cell membrane
   d. Include bacteria and Archaea

3. The primary structural difference between the prokaryote and eukaryote is _____.
   a. Prokaryotes are more like human cells.
   b. Prokaryotes have a semipermeable cell membrane.
   c. Prokaryotes have no distinct nucleus.
   d. Eukaryotes are not pathogenic.

4. The _____ protects the cell from drying and provides resistance to chemicals and invasion by viruses.
   a. Cell wall
   b. Capsule
   c. Cell membrane
   d. Spores

5. The _____ is also called the slime layer.
   a. Cell wall
   b. Cell membrane
   c. Outside layer of the nucleus
   d. Capsule

6. _____ is a process in which particles are engulfed.
   a. Phagocytosis
   b. Pinocytosis
   c. Active transport
   d. Endocytosis

7. The human intestinal tract contains many different types of bacteria, such as *Escherichia coli,* which are essential for digestion. This is an example of
_____ .
   a. Mutualism
   b. Parasitism
   c. Symbiosis
   d. Commensalism

8. What is the most effective way of controlling cross contamination in the health facility environment?
   a. Hand washing
   b. Sterilization of instruments before surgery.
   c. Keeping patient rooms clean
   d. Providing lockers for each employee

9. In the _____ phase symptoms begin to appear.
   a. Incubation
   b. Prodromal phase
   c. Acute phase
   d. Convalescence

10. In the _____ phase the organism is at its most potent.
   a. Incubation
   b. Prodromal phase
   c. Acute phase
   d. Convalescence

11. In the _____ phase the pathogens actively replicate.
   a. Incubation
   b. Prodromal phase
   c. Acute phase
   d. Convalescence

12. During the _____ phase, proliferation of the infectious organism slows and symptoms subside.
   a. Incubation
   b. Prodromal phase
   c. Acute phase
   d. Convalescence

13. The prion diseases are very significant in the surgical setting because
   a. They spread rapidly
   b. All surgical patients are at risk
   c. It is impossible to know who is a carrier
   d. They are resistant to all usual methods of destruction

14. Skin and mucous membrane are considered the first line of defense against disease because _____.
   a. Skin can be sterilized using disinfectants
   b. Once the skin is broken, infection can develop
   c. Skin contains many blood vessels
   d. Skin is very strong

15. Which surgical wound is associated with a higher risk of infection in the postoperative patient?
   a. Clean
   b. Clean-contaminated
   c. Contaminated
   d. All the above

16. The cardinal signs of inflammation are _____.
   a. Heat, redness, pain, swelling
   b. Pus, pain, redness, swelling
   c. Heat, pus, fever, pain
   d. Both A & C

17. Surgical site infection begins when a pathogenic or nonpathogenic microorganism colonizes sterile tissues. This can be caused by:
   a. Contamination of the tissues, such as a ruptured bowel or a traumatic wound caused by a foreign object.
   b. External contamination of the wound during convalescence.
   c. Poor surgical technique
   d. All of the above

18. Bacteria that causes infection is called _____.
   a. Contagious
   b. Toxic
   c. Pyogenic
   d. None of the above

19. Surgical site infection represents the
   a. greatest cause of hospital acquired infection
   b. the second most common cause of hospital acquired infection
   c. the most avoidable cause of hospital acquired infection
   d. the main reason for a hospital to loose accreditation

20. Bacteria require basic elemental nutrients, *except:*
   a. Oxygen
   b. Sulfur
   c. Water
   d. Carbon

21. All of the following are Gram positive bacteria, *except:*
   a. *Staphylococcus epidermidis*
   b. *Streptococcus Pyogenes*
   c. Gonorrhea
   d. *Streptococcus Pneumoniae*

22. A _____ is a nonliving infectious agent that ranges in size from 10 to 300 nm.
   a. Bacterium
   b. Virus
   c. Fungi
   d. Prion

23. The _____ is a unique pathogenic substance.
    a. Bacteria
    b. Virus
    c. Fungi
    d. Prion

24. _____ are found worldwide on living organic substances, in water, and in soil.
    a. Bacteria
    b. Virus
    c. Fungi
    d. Prion

25. _____ are a group of single-cell eukaryotic organisms.
    a. Protozoa
    b. Virus
    c. Fungi
    d. Algae

26. _____ are eukaryotes that belong to the plant kingdom; they include sponges and seaweed.
    a. Protozoa
    b. Virus
    c. Fungi
    d. Algae

27. _____ exists from the time of birth.
    a. Innate immunity
    b. Adaptive immunity

28. _____ conferred through exposure to a specific substance or microbe called an *antigen*.
    a. Innate immunity
    b. Adaptive immunity

29. _____ develops when the body receives the specific disease antibodies from an outside source.
    a. Active immunity
    b. Passive immunity
    c. Vaccination
    d. Hypersensitivity

30. Immune response to a substance is referred to as _____.
    a. Active
    b. Passive
    c. Vaccines
    d. Hypersensitivity

31. _____ is a process mediated by the immune system.
    a. True allergy
    b. Passive
    c. Vaccines
    d. Hypersensitivity

32. In certain diseases, the body does not recognize "self." This is known as _____.
    a. True allergy
    b. Autoimmunity
    c. Vaccines
    d. Hypersensitivity

33. There are two types of true allergic reactions:
    a. Immediate and reaction
    b. Reaction and delayed
    c. Delayed and immediate
    d. Immediate and true

1. *Read the following case study and answer the questions based on your knowledge of classification of surgical wounds:*

   You are scheduled for trauma call, and you get called in for a patient who was performing in a rodeo. He fell off his horse and is being admitted for an open fracture of the femur.

   a. How would this be classified?

   b. What is this patient's risk for infection?

   c. If the wound were not open and the patient were admitted for a femoral fracture, how would the wound be classified?

2. *Read the following case study and answer the questions based on your knowledge of identification of microorganisms.*

   You are in the operating room and scrubbed in. After entering the peritoneal cavity the surgeon finds free fluid in the abdomen, revealing an obvious infection. The surgeon asks for a culture. Answer the following questions about this case.

   a. What equipment and supplies do you request from your circulator?

b. What tests or examinations is the surgeon most likely to order for this case?

c. What tests or examinations are available from which the surgeon can choose?

d. Which test will the surgeon request if he or she wants or needs an immediate answer so that patient can be treated?

10 The Principles and Practice of Aseptic Technique

Student's Name_____

KEY TERMS

Write the definition for each term.

1. Antiseptics: _____

2. Asepsis: _____

3. Aseptic technique: _____

4. Chemical barrier: _____

5. Containment and confinement: _____

6. Contamination: _____

7. Double gloving: _____

8. Gross contamination: _____

9. Hand washing: _____

10. Nonsterile personnel: _____

11. Physical barrier: _____

12. Resident flora: _____

13. Scrub: _____

14. Scrubbed personnel: _____

15. Sharps: _____

16. Sterile field: _____

17. Sterile item: _____

18. Sterility: _____

19. Strike-through contamination: _____

20. Surgical conscience: _____

21. Surgical hand scrub: _____

22. Surgical handrub: _____

23. Surgical site infection (SSI): _____

24. Surgical wound: _____

25. Transient flora: _____

SHORT ANSWERS

Provide a short answer for each question or statement.

1. What are the four objectives of aseptic technique discussed in the text?

   a.

   b.

   c.

   d.

2. Where is the sterile field? What is the center of this area?

   _____

   _____

3. The methods used to achieve the goal of asepsis are called _____.

4. Items exposed (opened) to the surgical field are considered _____ after they
   have been exposed to the air or to a patient's tissues.

5. Sterile objects are contained or confined to avoid contact with _____ objects.

6. If any doubt exists about the sterility of an item, it should be considered _____.

7. Describe when a surgical technologist might choose to use a bouffant cap or a surgeon's cap.

   _____

   _____

   _____

8. The primary purpose of shoe covers is to _____.

74

Chapter **10 The Principles and Practice of Aseptic Technique**   Copyright © 2013, 2010, 2005 by Saunders, an imprint of Elsevier Inc.

9. _____, _____ and _____ are the three types of hand hygiene practiced in the operating room.

10. Masks must be worn in all restricted areas of the operating room. They should not be worn dangling around the neck *at any time* because _____

_____

_____

11. Home laundered head caps are not sanctioned by any infection control agency because _____

_____

_____

12. The surgical handrub is performed in place of a traditional surgical scrub *except when* _____

_____

_____

13. The traditional surgical scrub is performed in place of the handrub following _____

_____

_____

14. Sterile gowning and gloving takes place immediately after _____

_____

_____

15. The sterile towel, gown, and gloves should be opened on a clean surface away from where sterile instruments and other equipment has been opened to prevent _____

_____

_____

16. A gown should be changed during surgery if _____

_____

_____

17. Double gloving is perferred over single gloving because

_____

_____

18. Closed gloving technique is used when

_____

_____

19. Open gloving technique is used for

_____

_____

20. When gloving another person, you should open the glove, grasp the upper edges and offer it with the palm of the glove facing _____

_____

_____

21. If a surgical team member contaminates their glove during surgery, the circulator will remove it. This is done by offering the contaminated hand with the palm facing _____

_____

_____

MATCHING

Match each term with the correct definition.

1. _____ The application of an approved antiseptic to all surfaces of the hands and fingers

2. _____ A process meant to reduce the number of microorganisms on the skin to an absolute minimum

3. _____ Can be timed

4. _____ Counted strokes

5. _____ Ethyl or isopropyl alcohol combined with skin emollients

6. _____ Should be used only when no soil is visible on the hands

7. _____ Brushes must be sterile

8. _____ Event related

a. The principles of aseptic technique

b. Surgical scrub

c. Surgical rub

MATCHING

Match each term with the correct definition.

1. _____ are made of a lint-free synthetic material that is woven loosely enough to allow the breath to pass through effectively but tightly enough to filter 99% of particles of 5 micrograms or larger.

2. _____ are often worn by nonsterile perioperative personnel, for comfort and to prevent contamination of the surgical field through bacterial shedding from the arms.

3. _____ of any kind is a potential source of pathogens.

4. _____ are worn to reduce contamination of the surgical field by loose hair and dandruff from the scalp.

5. Perioperative personnel should wear _____ that are comfortable and easy to keep clean and that protect the wearer against foot injury.

6. _____ are worn any time surgical staff leave the department temporarily.

7. OSHA mandates the use of _____ or _____ as part of its blood-borne pathogen standard to protect workers exposed to splashing by blood and other potentially infectious materials (OPIM).

8. The _____ is designed to prevent the shedding of skin particles and hair into the environment and to protect the wearer from contact with soil and body fluids.

a. Protective eyewear/face shield

b. Head coverings

c. Jewelry

d. Scrub suit

e. Cover gowns/Lab coats

f. Non-sterile jackets

g. Masks

h. Shoes and covers

MULTIPLE CHOICE

Choose the most correct answer to the question or statement.

1. Which of the following is *not* an example of EBP?
   a. Double gloving
   b. Surgical hand scrub
   c. Surgical hand rub
   d. Lab coat
   e. Patient surgical site scrub

2. After an item has been sterilized, its sterility is maintained by _____.
   a. Surgical technologists
   b. Asepsis
   c. Decontamination
   d. Aseptic technique

3. The ethical and professional motivation that regulates a professional's behavior regarding disease transmission is known as _____.
   a. Tort
   b. Surgical law
   c. Surgical conscience
   d. Asepsis

4. A scrub suit must be changed if it:
   a. Is contaminated by blood or body fluid
   b. Comes in contact with the patient
   c. Comes in contact with any nonsterile item

5. Long-sleeved cover jackets are worn by the _____.
   a. Surgeon
   b. Scrub
   c. Circulator
   d. All of the above

6. At the end of the shift, the surgical technologist may place the scrub suit in his or her locker if:
   a. It is unsoiled.
   b. It does not have gross contaminants on it.
   c. The surgical technologist has worked less than 8 hours in it.
   d. The surgical technologist must never place the scrub suit in their locker at the end of a shift.

Chapter **10** **The Principles and Practice of Aseptic Technique**

7. When changing from street clothes to a scrub suit for entering the operating room, the surgical technologist puts on which of the following items first?
   a. Scrub pants
   b. Shoe covers
   c. Scrub shirt
   d. Head covering

8. The term for the area under the fingernails is _____.
   a. Sublingual
   b. Subungual
   c. Buccal
   d. Ungal

9. In the surgical scrub, which of the following comes first?
   a. Scrubbing the forearms
   b. Scrubbing the fingers
   c. Scrubbing the nail beds
   d. Applying the soap from fingers to elbows to "wash" the hands and arms

10. The surgical scrub extends to:
    a. 2 inches above the elbows
    b. The elbows
    c. Just below the elbows

11. When sterile supplies have been opened, the sterile setup is vulnerable to contamination. Once the sterile supplies have been opened, (select all that apply):
    a. They remain sterile for one hour.
    b. You must tape the OR door closed.
    c. They remain sterile for two hours.
    d. They must be continuously monitored to ensure sterility.

12. _____ is a way of making decisions and acting on proven methods.
    a. Evidence-based practice
    b. Surgical conscience
    c. Asepsis
    d. Aseptic technique

13. _____ is based on surgical conscience: that is, the ethical and professional motivation that regulates a professional's behaviors regarding disease transmission.
    a. Evidence-based practice
    b. Law
    c. Asepsis
    d. Aseptic technique

14. _____ occurs when the surgeon's gloved hand accidently touches the nonsterile edge of the surgical drape.
    a. Contamination
    b. A surgical error
    c. Antisepsis
    d. Aseptic technique

15. The _____ is worn by both sterile and nonsterile surgical personnel in the perioperative environment.
    a. Scrub suit
    b. Body lotion
    c. Leather shoes
    d. Lab coat

16. At the close of the case, gown and gloves are removed:
    a. By pulling gloves off first
    b. By removing the gown first and then gloves
    c. By breaking all the ties with gloved hands after removing gloves
    d. By pulling from the back

17. Before opening a sterile pack, the scrub should also check the outside package for the:
    a. Right size
    b. Integrity
    c. Right wrap
    d. Colored tape

18. What operating room furniture should the large pack be placed on before opening?
    a. Ring stand
    b. Mayo stand
    c. Back table
    d. Prep stand

19. What operating room furniture should the instrument tray be placed on prior to opening?
    a. Ring stand
    b. Mayo stand
    c. Back table
    d. Prep stand

20. What operating room furniture should the basin set be placed on before opening?
    a. Ring stand
    b. Mayo stand
    c. Back table
    d. Prep stand

21. Items wrapped in _____ are delivered directly to the scrub by grasping the top edges of the wrapper and peeling the wrapper apart to reveal the sterile item.
   a. Sterile wrap
   b. Sealed pouches
   c. Sealed wrap
   d. Original package

22. All of the following are correct about pouring solution on the sterile field, *except:*
   a. The lip of a solution bottle is considered sterile only if it is covered with a sterile top that extends over the edge of the container.
   b. The recommended method of distributing a solution is to pour the solution directly into a container set close to the edge of the table or held in the hand of the scrub.
   c. When pouring sterile liquids, do not empty the entire container and move the downturned container away from the sterile field.
   d. Never remove the cap of a medicine vial using an instrument and then pour out the contents.

CASE STUDIES

1. *Read the following case study and answer the questions about opening a sterile table.*

   Look at the picture and answer the following questions about the actions of the surgical technologist.

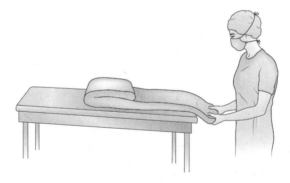

   a. The surgical technologist has just opened one side of her sterile table. What are her next three actions? (Be specific.)

2. *Answer the following questions about evidence-based practice.*

    a. What is evidence-based practice?

    b. Why is it so important to the surgical technologist?

    c. How can you practice evidence-based practice every day?

    d. Who is responsible for ensuring that EBP is being conducted?

11 Decontamination, Sterilization, and Disinfection

Student's Name _____

KEY TERMS

Write the definition for each term.

1. Association for the Advancement of Medical Instrumentation (AAMI): _____

2. Antisepsis _____

4. Bactericidal _____

5. Bacteriostatic _____

6. Biofilms _____

7. Biological indicators _____

8. Case cart system _____

9. Cavitation _____

10. Central service department _____

11. Central processing technician _____

12. Chemical indicator _____

13. Chemical sterilization _____

14. –cidal _____

15. Cleaning _____

16. Cobalt 60 radiation _____

17. Contaminated _____

18. Decontamination _____

19. Detergent _____

20. Disinfection _____

21. Enzymatic cleaner _____

22. Ethylene oxide (EO) _____

23. Event-related sterility _____

24. Evidence-based practices _____

25. Exposure time _____

26. Fungicidal _____

27. Gas plasma sterilization _____

28. Germicidal _____

29. Gravity displacement sterilizer _____

30. High level disinfection (HLD) _____

31. High-vacuum sterilizer _____

32. Inanimate _____

33. Implant _____

34. Immediate-use sterilization _____

35. International Association of Healthcare Central Service Material Management (IAHCSMM) _____

36. Material Safety Data Sheets _____

37. Medical device _____

38. Noncritical items _____

39. Nonwoven _____

40. Peracetic acid _____

41. Personal protective equipment (PPE) _____

42. Prion _____

43. Process challenge monitoring _____

44. Reprocessing _____

45. Reusable _____

46. Sanitation _____

47. Sharps _____

48. Shelf life _____

49. Single-use items _____

50. Spaulding system _____

51. Sporicidal _____

52. Sterilization _____

53. Terminal decontamination _____

54. Ultrasonic cleaner _____

55. Virucidal _____

56. Washer-sterilizer/decontaminator _____

57. Woven wrappers _____

SHORT ANSWERS

Provide a short answer for each question or statement.

1. Before the washer-sterilizer cycle is finished, the instruments are considered _____. What is the purpose of the washer-sterilizer?

   _____

   _____

2. After the instruments are taken to the clean assembly area, what are the next steps for?

   _____

   _____

3. Items with a lumen should have a small amount of _____ flushed through them immediately before sterilization.

   _____

   _____

MATCHING

Match each term with the correct definition. Some terms may be used more than once.

1. _____ Provides recommended practices and technical information for U.S. medical professions

2. _____ Accreditation agency for all health care organizations in the United States

3. _____ Professional association for perioperative nurses

4. _____ An organization for which standards are developed with the support of the U.S. Food and Drug Administration

5. _____ Agency of the federal government that provides research and protocols in all areas of public health

6. _____ Organization that oversees compliance with environmental and patient safety regulations

a. AAMI
b. AORN
c. CDC
d. TJC

Choose the most correct answer to complete the question.

1. _____ is a chemical used to remove micro-organisms on tissue.
   a. An antiseptic
   b. A disinfectant
   c. Sterilization
   d. All of the above

2. The system that assigns a device a risk category based on the specific regions of the body where the device is used is the _____ system.
   a. Spaulding
   b. Sterilization
   c. Dewey
   d. Maslow

3. Which of the following body tissues presents a critical risk in the Spaulding system?
   a. Hands
   b. Intact skin
   c. Vascular system
   d. Mucosal membranes

4. _____ is a skilled, certified profession requiring expertise in the science and practice of materials management, decontamination, and sterilization.
   a. Perioperative nursing
   b. Anesthesiology
   c. Central processing
   d. Certified nurse's aides

5. The _____ is used to transport sterile and nonsterile instruments and equipment to and from the main operating room area.
   a. Crash cart
   b. Elevator
   c. Case cart

6. The washer-sterilizer or washer-disinfector is used to process all instruments that can tolerate
   a. Heat
   b. Water turbulence and high pressure steam
   c. Strong disinfectant
   d. Cold solutions

7. The _____ includes a workroom with ample table space for sorting instruments and assembling instrument sets.
   a. Clean processing area
   b. Decontamination area
   c. Sterile back table
   d. Case cart system

8. Instruments that have _____ must be disassembled before sterilization.
   a. Removable parts
   b. Ratchets
   c. Sharp edges
   d. Blades

9. Instrument trays have a perforated bottom so that:
   a. Steam can circulate up through the tray and adequately cover all surfaces of the instruments.
   b. They are easier for the surgical team to handle.
   c. The instruments are easily put into sets by central processing.
   d. The towels in the instrument sets cannot be damaged by the steam.

10. Which of the following statements is *not* true regarding the use of peel pouches?
    a. Items wrapped in peel pouches must not be placed inside an instrument tray.
    b. Double pouches are unnecessary and may prevent sterilization of the item.
    c. The item in the pouch should clear the seal by at least 1 inch.
    d. Peel pouches are intended for items such as bone rongeurs, rasps, and multiple instruments.

11. Which type of sterilization method requires an aeration?
    a. Steam
    b. Steam under pressure
    c. Ethylene oxide
    d. Gas plasma

12. Which of the following sterilizers uses peracetic acid?
    a. Steris
    b. Flash
    c. Ethylene oxide
    d. Gas plasma

13. Which of the following high level disinfectants could also be used as a sterilizing agent?
    a. Gas plasma
    b. Peracetic acid
    c. Glutaraldehyde
    d. Steam

14. The following are high level disinfection semi-critical items, *except:*
    a. Operating room table and accessories
    b. Respiratory therapy equipment
    c. Bronchoscopes
    d. Anesthesia equipment

15. The following are low level disinfection noncritical items, *except:*
    a. Operating room table and accessories
    b. Furniture in the surgical suite
    c. Bronchoscopes
    d. Blood pressure cuffs

CASE STUDIES

1. *Read the following case study and answer the following questions.*

   You are scrubbed into an emergency case involving a patient with a fractured hip. The instruments that your hospital uses to repair the fracture were used earlier in the day and are not sterile. The set includes the implants. You put the instruments in the flash sterilizer:

   a. Define flash sterilization.

   b. Can you run implants through the flash sterilization process? Explain.

   c. At what temperature did you run the implants?

   d. For how many minutes did you set the autoclave to run?

Chapter **11** Decontamination, Sterilization, and Disinfection

e. How do you know the instruments have been through the sterilization process when you retrieve them?

f. When flashing implants, what indicator is to be included with the implants?

g. How long after flashing implants can they be cleared for use?

2. *Read the following case study and answer the following questions.*

You are scrubbed into a case where the patient has an infection in his hip. The surgeon wants to take the implant out and "flash" it, you ask the instrument room coordinator and she asks the following question:

a. Why can't you use another implant?

b. How long must you wait for an implant to be sterilized before going back into the patient?

c. What other options does the surgeon have if the implant cannot be sterilized?

d. What problems will the patient have if the implant comes back positive?

3. *Answer the questions below about CJD:*

   a. What are prions?

   b. What causes CJD?

c. Why is CJD a concern with regard to sterilization methods?

d. What are the AAMI guidelines to prevent TASS?

12 Surgical Instruments

Student's Name _____

KEY TERMS

Write the definition for each term.

1. Alloy: _____

2. Box lock: _____

3. Chisel: _____

4. Curettage: _____

5. Dilator: _____

6. Double-action instrument: _____

7. Elevator: _____

8. Gouge: _____

9. Hemostat: _____

10. Rongeur: _____

11. Serosa: _____

12. Shank: _____

13. Single action rongeur: _____

14. Tenaculum: _____

LABELING

Label the following diagram of a locking clamp.

1.

2.

3.

4.

5.

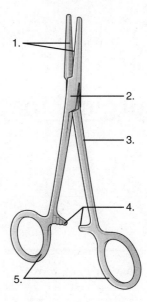

MATCHING

Match each instrument with its classification (One or more choices may not be used.)

1. _____ Crile
2. _____ Allis
3. _____ Babcock
4. _____ Adson forceps
5. _____ Frazier
6. _____ Army/Navy
7. _____ Curved Mayo
8. _____ Key elevator
9. _____ Kerrison or Pituitary
10. _____ Sweetheart
11. _____ Webster
12. _____ Sims uterine sound
13. _____ Mayo-Hegar
14. _____ GIA
15. _____ LDS
16. _____ Yankauer
17. _____ Clip applier
18. _____ Duvall lung clamp
19. _____ Richardson Eastman
20. _____ Metz
21. _____ Sterile ruler
22. _____ Mosquito
23. _____ Kocher/Oschner
24. _____ DeBakey forceps
25. _____ Balfour
26. _____ #3 knife handle
27. _____ Curved iris

a. Cutting
b. Clamping
c. Grasping
d. Suturing
e. Dilating
f. Measuring
g. Stapling
h. Retracting
i. Suction
j. Hemostatic clips

MATCHING

Match the correct knife handle with the correct blade.

1. _____ Round   a. # 3 Short
2. _____ # 10   b. # 3 Long
3. _____ # 11   c. # 7
4. _____ # 12   d. #. 4 Short
5. _____ # 15   e. #. 4 Long
6. _____ # 20   f. # 9
7. _____ Chisel   g. Beaver
8. _____ Curved
9. _____ # 25
10. _____ # 23

SHORT ANSWERS

Provide a short answer for each question or statement.

1. Explain the difference in a self-retaining retractor and a handheld retractor. Also, give an example of each and the surgical procedure for which you would use the retractor.

_____

_____

2. What is the name of the instrument used to measure the depth of the uterus?

_____

_____

3. You are the scrub for an exploratory laparotomy, where the surgeon is irrigating the abdomen. What suction tip would you use and why?

_____

_____

4. You are the second circulator in the room and the circulator asks you to get an EEA stapler. What surgical procedure would you use the stapler for?

_____

_____

5. You are scrubbed in on a liver resection and the surgeon asks for forceps. What type of forceps would you use and why?

_____

_____

6. You are scrubbed on an ORIF of the ankle, and the surgeon asks for an elevator. What type of elevator would you use and why?

_____

_____

7. During a TURP, the surgeon asks for an instrument to open the stricture of the urethra. What type of instrument would you give the surgeon?

_____

_____

8. You are scrubbed on a thyroidectomy and the surgeon asks for a clip. What type would you give the surgeon and why?

_____

_____

9. You are scrubbed on a total knee arthroplasty and the surgeon asks for an instrument to scrape out a portion of diseased bone. What type of instrument would you give the surgeon?

_____

_____

10. You are scrubbed on a laparoscopic cholecystectomy and the surgeon asks for a hemostat. What type of hemostat would you give the surgeon and why?

_____

_____

11. The surgeon is closing the skin. What type of forceps would the surgeon use and why?

_____

_____

MULTIPLE CHOICE

Choose the correct answer for each question.

1. An example of an angled instrument is a(n) _____.
   a. Schnidt
   b. Right angle
   c. Osteotome
   d. Deaver

2. Which instrument penetrates the tissue rather than just holding it?
   a. Tenaculum
   b. Babcock
   c. Kelly
   d. Lowman

3. Which instrument is used to grasp the fallopian tube or intestinal tissue?
   a. Allis clamp
   b. Babcock clamp
   c. Kelly hemostat
   d. Pean

4. All of the following are types of elevators, *except:*
   a. Cushing joker
   b. Cup curette
   c. Cob elevator
   d. Key elevator

5. Which instrument is used to remove bone using a biting action?
   a. Rongeur
   b. Osteotome
   c. Curette
   d. Shears

6. Which instrument is used to remove excess fluid from the throat?
   a. Poole suction tip
   b. Yankauer suction tip
   c. Frazier suction tip
   d. Joseph suction tip

7. Choose the self-retaining retractor that is used during open heart surgery.
   a. Finochietto
   b. Balfour
   c. Gelpi
   d. Weitlaner

8. Which instrument is used to retract vessels during surgery?
   a. Army-Navy retractor
   b. Cushing vein retractor
   c. Goelet retractor
   d. Richardson retractor

9. What classification is a tenotomy?
   a. Retractor
   b. Cutting
   c. Forceps
   d. Miscellaneous

10. All the following instruments can be used in an amputation, *except:*
    a. #4 knife handle
    b. Mayo scissors
    c. Metzenbaum scissors
    d. Babcock clamp

11. Which instrument is used in nasal procedures?
    a. Babcock clamp
    b. Bayonet forceps
    c. Double-tooth tenaculum
    d. Mayo scissors

12. Which instrument is used to clamp small blood vessels?
    a. Babcock clamp
    b. Duval lung clamp
    c. Mosquito hemostat
    d. Crile hemostat

13. What classification is a Kocher? Select all that apply.
    a. Clamping
    b. Grasping
    c. Retracting
    d. Cutting

14. What classification is a Babcock? Select all that apply.
    a. Clamping
    b. Grasping
    c. Retracting
    d. Cutting

15. What classification is a hemostat?
    a. Clamping
    b. Grasping
    c. Retracting
    d. Cutting

16. What classification is a Richardson Eastman?
    a. Clamping
    b. Grasping
    c. Retracting
    d. Cutting

17. What type of tissue would a Heaney needle holder be used for?
    a. Dura mater
    b. Sclera
    c. Blood vessel
    d. Uterus

18. The surgeon is working on the bowel. He is dissecting the omentum and needs a clamp. What clamp would he need?
    a. Crile
    b. Tonsil
    c. Kelly
    d. Babcock

19. _____ reduces glare but is also prone to staining.
    a. Highly polished or mirror finish
    b. Satin finish
    c. Black chromium
    d. Titanium anodizing

20. _____ instruments resist staining.
   a. Highly polished or mirror finish
   b. Satin finish
   c. Black chromium
   d. Titanium anodizing

21. _____ is a finishing method that imparts color and hardness to the surface of titanium.
   a. Highly polished or mirror
   b. Satin
   c. Black chromium
   d. Titanium anodizing

22. _____ finish is used on laser surgery instruments.
   a. Highly polished or mirror finish
   b. Satin
   c. Black chromium
   d. Titanium anodizing

23. The _____ is a small cup with a sharpened, serrated, or smooth rim at the end of the handle.
   a. Rongeur
   b. Osteotome
   c. Curette
   d. Shears

24. A _____ is a V-shaped bone chisel.
   a. Rongeur
   b. Osteotome
   c. Curette
   d. Gouge

25. A _____ is used to remodel bone.
   a. Rasp
   b. Curette
   c. Chisel
   d. Osteotome

CASE STUDIES

1. *Read the following case study and answer the questions based on your knowledge of surgical instruments.*

   You are scrubbed in on a vascular case, and your surgeon is about to make an incision into the carotid artery. He will need several instruments in sequence. Using your critical thinking skills, answer the following questions about the instruments.

   a. What scalpel blade will your surgeon most likely use to make the incision into the artery?

   b. What instrument will the surgeon need the very second the incision is made?

   c. What instrument will the surgeon use to retract the tissue?

d. What scissors will the surgeon use on the soft tissue?

e. What instrument will the surgeon use to clamp the small vessels?

2. *Briefly describe the following surgical instruments. Be sure to include the materials of which they are made and the purposes for which they are used.*

   a. Surgical-grade instruments

   b. Bright (or mirror) finish instruments

   c. Satin finish instruments

d. Ebony finish instruments

e. Disposable instruments

Student's Name: _____ Date: _____

Task: Student will identify the proper instruments and the classification.

Equipment and Supplies: Have available one instrument from each classification.

Evaluation Directions: Check or circle the appropriate number to indicate the student's performance level, using the following rating scale:

3-PROFICIENT. Can complete the task quickly and accurately without direction.

2-PARTIALLY PROFICIENT. Can do most of the task. Needs assistance. Needs constant supervision.

1-LIMITED. Can do a limited amount of the task. Must be told what to do. Needs extremely close supervision.

0-UNSATISFACTORY. Can do a limited amount of the task. Must be told what to do. Needs extremely close supervision.

Task Checklist	Rating	Self-Assessment	Instructor Assessment
1. Identify instruments in each classification			
a. Accessory	0 1 2 3		
b. Aspirating and suctioning	0 1 2 3		
c. Clamping/occluding	0 1 2 3		
d. Cutting/dissecting	0 1 2 3		
e. Dilating	0 1 2 3		
f. Grasping/holding	0 1 2 3		
g. Probing	0 1 2 3		
h. Retracting/exposing	0 1 2 3		
i. Suturing	0 1 2 3		
j. Stapling	0 1 2 3		
2. Care and handling			
a. Checking function and integrity	0 1 2 3		
b. Cleaning methods	0 1 2 3		
c. Terminal sterilization	0 1 2 3		
d. Lubrication	0 1 2 3		
e. Preparation for sterilization	0 1 2 3		
f. Safety precautions	0 1 2 3		

Task Checklist	Rating	Self-Assessment	Instructor Assessment
3. Assembling sets			
a. Types of sets	0 1 2 3		
b. Types of instrument trays, pans, and container systems	0 1 2 3		
c. Instrument checklist (count sheet)	0 1 2 3		
d. Techniques of assembly	0 1 2 3		
Total Score			

SCORE

60-54 = A

53-48 = B

47-42 = C

Below 42 = not passing

Comments:

_____

_____

_____

_____

13 Perioperative Pharmacology

Student's Name _____

KEY TERMS

Write the definition for each term.

1. Adverse reaction: _____.

2. Agonist: _____.

3. Allergy: _____.

4. Antagonist: _____.

5. Antibiotics: _____.

6. Bioavailability: _____.

7. Chemical name: _____.

8. Concentration: _____.

9. Contraindication: _____.

10. Contrast media: _____.

11. Controlled substances: _____.

12. Diluent: _____.

13. Dosage: _____.

14. Dose: _____.

15. Drug: _____.

16. Drug administration: _____.

17. Generation: _____.

18. Generic name: _____.

19. Half-life: _____.

20. Hypersensitivity: _____.

21. Intraosseous: _____.

22. Intrathecal: _____.

23. Parenteral: _____.

24. Peak effect: _____.

25. Pharmacodynamics: _____.

26. Pharmacokinetics: _____.

27. Pharmacology: _____.

28. Prescription: _____.

29. Proprietary name: _____.

30. Side effects: _____.

31. Therapeutic window: _____.

32. Topical: _____.

33. Trade name: _____.

34. Transdermal: _____.

35. U.S. Pharmacopeia (USP): _____.

SHORT ANSWERS

Provide a short answer for each question or statement.

1. Drugs used in modern medicine are derived from a number of sources. Name the sources, and give an example of each.

   _____

   _____

2. The Joint Commission (TJC) requires health care organizations develop policies that agree with state laws regulating who may handle drugs and in what circumstances. What activities must be regulated?

   _____

   _____

3. List 5 of the 26 dosage forms and define.

   _____

   _____

4. Describe the medication process.

_____

_____

5. The FDA maintains strict regulatory control on devices and substances used on or in the body, this includes:

_____

_____

6. List the four types of allergic reactions, and explain the differences between them.

a. _____

b. _____

c. _____

d. _____

7. Who or what indicates or recommends a route for drug administration to a patient?

_____

_____

8. If you are scrubbed and you are about to label the medication on your table, what information must be on the label?

_____

_____

9. In Roman numerals, give the year in which you will graduate from your surgical technology program.

_____

_____

10. List the 10 elements that have the most influence on drug errors.

a. _____

b. _____

c. _____

d. _____

e. _____

f. _____

g. _____

h. _____

i. _____

j. _____

11. What are the three commonly used staining solutions and what are they used for during the intraoperative period?

a. _____

b. _____

c. _____

12. When are topical antibiotics used for wound irrigation?

_____

_____

13. What is the difference between a staining agent, a dye, and a contrast medium?

_____

_____

14. What is the difference between colloids and crystalloids? Give an example of each.

a. Example of a colloid:

_____

b. Example of a crystal:

_____

15. List the seven drug rights and define.

a. _____

b. _____

c. _____

d. _____

e. _____

f. _____

g. _____

16. List the elements of a prescription.

_____

_____

17. List different types of medication orders and define.

_____

_____

18. List the protocol for receiving and dispensing drugs on the sterile field.

_____

_____

19. What time is 2:10 PM in military time?

_____

_____

20. Using the following drug label, answer these questions:

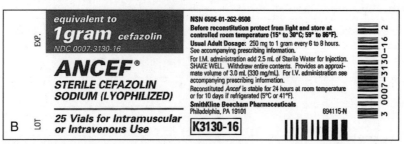

From Kee J, Hayes E, McCuiston L: *Pharmacology*, ed 5, Philadelphia, 2006, WB Saunders.

a. What is the generic name?

_____

_____

b. What is the *proprietary* name?

_____

_____

c. What is the dosage form?

_____

_____

d. What is the dosage and route of administration?

_____

_____

e. What are the contraindications?

_____

_____

MATCHING

Match each term with the correct definition.

1. _____ Is the complete reference of all drugs, dietary supplements, and devices marketed for medical use in the United States

2. _____ Research drugs using the Internet

3. _____ Is used by many primary health care providers

4. _____ A number of products related to safe use of drugs

a. The Physicians' Desk Reference (PDR)

b. The United States Pharmacopeia-National Formulary (USP-NF)

c. The American Hospital Formulary Service

d. Online Drug Resources

MATCHING

Match each measurement with the correct name and number.

1. _____ = 1,000 meters

2. _____ = 1,000 grams

3. _____ = 1/1000 of a gram

4. _____ = 1/1000 of a liter

5. _____ = 5/1000 of a liter

6. _____ = 0.1 (one tenth)

7. _____ = 0.01 (one hundredth)

8. _____ = 0.001 (one thousandth)

9. _____ = 1,000 microliters

A. 5 *milli*liters

B. Deci

C. 1 *milli*gram

D. Centi

E. 1 *kilo*gram

F. Milli

G. 1 *kilo*meter

H. 1 *milli*liter

MATCHING

Match the route of administration with the dosage form.

1. _____ Sublingual

2. _____ Intravenous

3. _____ Vaginal

4. _____ Intraosseous (IO)

5. _____ Subcutaneous (SQ)

6. _____ Intradermal (ID)

7. _____ Transdermal

8. _____ Intraperitoneal

9. _____ Ingestion

10. _____ Inhalant

11. _____ Intramuscular (IM)

12. _____ Instillation

13. _____ Rectal

14. _____ Buccal

15. _____ Nasal

16. _____ Intraspinal

a. Parenteral

b. Oral

c. Topical

MULTIPLE CHOICE

Choose the most correct answer to complete the question or statement.

1. Drugs that enhance uterine contractions are called
   _____.
   a. Uterotropics
   b. Pitressin
   c. Synthroid
   d. Isoproterenol

2. In the United States, strict controls and standards
   are maintained for _____.
   a. All agents used in the body
   b. Only drugs
   c. Only artificial implants and medical devices
   d. Wound closure materials
   e. All of the above

3. Drugs that fall in _____ are determined
   to have no medical use.
   a. Schedule V
   b. Schedules III and IV
   c. Schedule II
   d. Schedule I

4. Drugs that are classified by pregnancy category include:
   a. A, Z, and X
   b. A, B, C, and X
   c. Schedules I, II, III, IV, and V
   d. None of the above

5. Most pregnancy category drugs are listed as
   _____ because it is unknown whether
   they pose a risk.
   a. Category A
   b. Schedule C
   c. Category D
   d. Schedule V

6. The route of a drug may not identify the drug's
   final destination. This statement is true of which
   of the following drugs?
   a. Injectable lidocaine
   b. IM Ancef
   c. Transdermal nitroglycerin
   d. IV heparin sodium

7. Which of the following medications can be administered intravenously?
   a. Gelfoam
   b. Heparin sodium
   c. Thrombin
   d. Bone wax

8. The action of a drug as it is broken down chemically
   is called _____.
   a. Passive diffusion
   b. Pharmacokinetics
   c. Pharmacodynamics
   d. Digestion

9. With regard to pharmacokinetics, which of the
   following processes might involve active transport?
   a. Absorption
   b. Distribution
   c. Metabolism
   d. Excretion

10. The _____ is the amount of time it takes
    for one half of the drug to be cleared from the body.
    a. Peak and trough
    b. Distribution
    c. Half-life
    d. Metabolism

11. Which of the following would be true when
    discussing a drug allergy?
    a. The drug/reaction elicits an immune system
       response.
    b. Drug allergies are a known effect that occurs in
       some patients.
    c. Drug allergies are treated locally and are rarely
       serious.
    d. Drug allergies always manifest themselves first
       by presenting with a rash.

12. Which of the following describes a type II drug
    allergy?
    a. Anaphylactic shock
    b. Hemolytic disease in newborns
    c. Allergy to antibiotics
    d. A positive reaction to the tuberculin skin test

13. The patient's weight is always calculated for
    _____.
    a. Pediatric patients
    b. Elderly patients
    c. Patients with diabetes
    d. Adolescents

14. Which of the following is *not* absorbed but is excreted through the GI tract?
    a. Lugol solution
    b. Methylene blue
    c. Barium
    d. Iodinated contrast medium

15. For what purpose are topical hemostatics used intraoperatively?
    a. To control bleeding from a small capillary complex
    b. To control massive hemorrhage
    c. To assist in the closure of the wound
    d. To promote healing and prevent the formation of a seroma

16. Which of the following is categorized as a topical anticoagulant?
    a. Thrombin
    b. Gelfoam
    c. Heparin sodium
    d. Ostene

17. _____ stimulate the responses of the sympathetic system.
    a. Cholinergics
    b. Antiadrenergics
    c. Adrenergics
    d. Anticholinergics

CASE STUDIES

1. *Read the following case study and answer the questions:*

   You have been asked to scrub up and open the room for a neurology case. Your circulator is busy finishing a case in another operating room. You want to make sure you have all the supplies you will need for the sterile field, as well as all the supplies your circulator will need. The surgeon's preference card asks for the following medications:

   - *1 g Ancef in 1,000 normal saline irrigation*

   - *5,000 units heparin sodium in 500 IV NaCl*

   - *Hypaque dye 20/20*

   - *0.25% lidocaine with 1:200,000 epinephrine*

   - *1 vial of methylene blue*

   a. What are your defined responsibilities in delivering the medication to the sterile field?

   b. The heparin sodium arrives from the pharmacy in a glass ampule. Are there any special instructions you should follow with this medication?

c. What method will you use to draw up the medication after you have scrubbed in?

2. *Read the following case study and answer the questions:*

Today you are helping in preoperative holding as an assistant circulator. Your patient, Mr. Buckner, has come down, and you are checking his vital signs. He is in preop holding waiting for his ankle arthroscopy to begin. Mr. Buckner tells you that he suddenly "does not feel very good." You notice that his face and neck are quite red compared to the rest of his body. You know that the RN in preop holding has just started an IV and administered Mr. Buckner's preop antibiotic. You have just recorded that Mr. Buckner's vital signs are:

Pulse: 102

Respirations: 14

Blood pressure: 140/74

Temperature: 37° C

Oxygen saturation: 97%

a. What signs do you observe that you believe are not normal for this patient?

b. What does the patient report suggest?

c. What does the patient report?

d. What comfort measures could you initiate?

e. Whom do you tell about the change in the patient's condition?

SKILLS PERFORMANCE CHECKLIST: DRAW UP MEDICATION IN A SYRINGE INTO THE STERILE FIELD

Student's Name: _____ Date: _____

Task: Student identifies proper medication and accepts medication onto sterile field.

Equipment and Supplies:

- Proper medication
- Alcohol prep
- Appropriate syringe and needle

Evaluation Directions: Check or circle the appropriate number to indicate the student's performance level, using the following rating scale:

3-PROFICIENT. Can complete the task quickly and accurately without direction.

2-PARTIALLY PROFICIENT. Can do most of the task. Needs assistance. Needs constant supervision.

1-LIMITED. Can do a limited amount of the task. Must be told what to do. Needs extremely close supervision.

0-UNSATISFACTORY. Can do a limited amount of the task. Must be told what to do. Needs extremely close supervision.

Task Checklist	Rating	Self-Assessment	Instructor Assessment
1. Verify patient allergies.	0 1 2 3		
2. Circulator prepares medication for withdrawal.	0 1 2 3		
3. STSR and circulator visually and verbally confirm correct medication.	0 1 2 3		
4. STSR withdraws medication from container using proper technique.	0 1 2 3		
5. STSR and circulator visually and verbally confirm correct medication.	0 1 2 3		
6. Medication is labeled on the field.	0 1 2 3		
7. Medication is passed to surgeon when requested and verbally identified.	0 1 2 3		
Total Score			

Chapter **13** **Perioperative Pharmacology**   Copyright © 2013, 2010, 2005 by Saunders, an imprint of Elsevier Inc.

SCORE

21-18 = A

17-13 = B

12-10 = C

Below 10 = not passing

Comments:

_____

_____

_____

_____

14 Anesthesia and Physiological Monitoring

Student's Name _____

Write the definition for each term.

1. Airway: _____

2. Amnesia: _____

3. Analgesia: _____

4. Anesthesia: _____

5. Anesthesia care provider (ACP): _____

6. Anesthesia machine: _____

7. Anesthesia technologist: _____

8. Anesthesiologist: _____

9. Anesthetic: _____

10. Antegrade amnesia: _____

11. Anxiolytic: _____

12. Apnea: _____

13. Bier block: _____

14. Bispectral index system (BIS): _____

15. Breathing bag: _____

16. Central nervous system depression: _____

17. Coma: _____

18. Consciousness: _____

19. Delirium: _____

20. Emergence: _____

21. Endotracheal tube: _____

22. Esmarch bandage: _____

23. Extubation: _____

24. Gas scavenging: _____

25. General anesthesia: _____

26. Homeostasis: _____

27. Hypothermia: _____

28. Induction: _____

29. Intraoperative awareness (IOA): _____

30. Intravascular volume: _____

31. Intubation: _____

32. Laryngeal mask airway (LMA): _____

33. Laryngoscope: _____

34. Malignant hyperthermia (MH): _____

35. Monitored anesthesia care (MAC): _____

36. Nasopharyngeal airway: _____

37. Neuromuscular blocking agent: _____

38. Oropharyngeal airway (OPA): _____

39. Perfusion: _____

40. Physiological monitoring: _____

41. Pneumatic tourniquet: _____

42. Postanesthesia recovery unit (PACU): _____

43. Preoperative medication: _____

44. Protective reflexes: _____

45. Pulmonary embolism (PE): _____

46. Pulse oximeter: _____

47. Regional block: _____

48. Sedation: _____

49. Sedative: _____

50. Sensation: _____

51. Topical anesthesia: _____

52. Unconsciousness: _____

53. Ventilation: _____

54. Vital signs: _____

LABELING

Label the laryngeal mask.

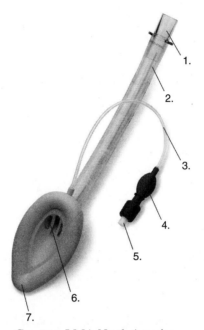

Courtesy LMA North America.

1.

2.

3.

4.

5.

6.

7.

Chapter **14** **Anesthesia and Physiological Monitoring**

SHORT ANSWERS

Provide a short answer for each question or statement.

1. Anesthesia means "without sensation." What is the goal of surgical anesthesia?

_____

_____

2. What are the eight senses?

   a.

   b.

   c.

   d.

   e.

   f.

   g.

   h.

3. List the primary goal of the ACP.

_____

_____

4. What seven things help the surgeon, the ACP, and the patient decide which type of anesthetic will be best for the individual during the procedure?

   a.

   b.

   c.

   d.

   e.

   f.

   g.

5. Hospitals and other surgical facilities have individual check-in protocols. Which specific details are always verified?

_____

_____

6. List the routine patient parameters that must be monitored and give an example of each.

_____

_____

7. What are the four phases of anesthesia?

a.

b.

c.

d.

MATCHING

Match each term with the correct definition.

1. _____ Intravascular monitoring
2. _____ Pulmonary artery catheter
3. _____ Capnography
4. _____ BUN
5. _____ ABG
6. _____ BIS
7. _____ Pulse oximetry
8. _____ Malignant hyperthermia
9. _____ Intravascular volume
10. _____ ECG
11. _____ Arterial blood pressure monitoring
12. _____ IOA
13. _____ Transesophageal monitoring
14. _____ 97° to 99.5° F
15. _____ Hypothermia
16. _____ Peripheral nerve stimulator

a. Ventilation
b. Perfusion
c. Fluid and electrolyte balance
d. Direct (invasive)
e. Indirect (noninvasive)
f. Renal failure
g. Body temperature
h. Neuromuscular response
i. Level of consciousness

Choose the most correct answer to complete the question or statement.

1. _____ is an invasive airway that extends from the mouth to the trachea.
   a. OPA (Oropharyngeal airway)
   b. LMA (Laryngeal mask airway)
   c. NPA (Nasopharyngeal airway)
   d. ET tube (Endotracheal tube)

2. _____ provides passage between the nostril and the nasopharynx.
   a. OPA (Oropharyngeal airway)
   b. LMA (Laryngeal mask airway)
   c. NPA (Nasopharyngeal airway)
   d. ET tube (Endotracheal tube)

3. _____ is inserted over the tongue to prevent the tongue or epiglottis from falling back against the pharynx.
   a. OPA (Oropharyngeal airway)
   b. LMA (Laryngeal mask airway)
   c. NPA (Nasopharyngeal airway)
   d. ET tube (Endotracheal tube)

4. _____ is inserted without the aid of a laryngoscope and fits snugly over the larynx.
   a. OPA (Oropharyngeal airway)
   b. LMA (Laryngeal mask airway)
   c. NPA (Nasopharyngeal airway)
   d. ET tube (Endotracheal tube)

5. The most crucial time for the patient with a difficult airway is during _____.
   a. Preop and postop
   b. Preop and extubation
   c. Intubation and postop
   d. Intubation and extubation

6. The _____ phase involves continuation of the anesthetic agent.
   a. Induction
   b. Maintenance
   c. Emergence
   d. Recovery

7. Post anesthesia care is provided in the _____ phase.
   a. Induction
   b. Maintenance
   c. Emergence
   d. Recovery

8. During the _____ phase, general anesthesia begins with loss of consciousness.
   a. Induction
   b. Maintenance
   c. Emergence
   d. Recovery

9. The _____ phase is the cessation of the anesthetic.
   a. Induction
   b. Maintenance
   c. Emergence
   d. Recovery

10. During _____ the patient is relaxed, and protective reflexes are lost.
    a. Stage 1
    b. Stage 2
    c. Stage 3
    d. Stage 4

11. _____ begins with the administration of induction drugs and ends with loss of consciousness.
    a. Stage 1
    b. Stage 2
    c. Stage 3
    d. Stage 4

12. During what stage can anesthesia overdose resulting in severe respiratory and circulatory collapse occur?
    a. Stage 1
    b. Stage 2
    c. Stage 3
    d. Stage 4

13. During _____, delirium ensues, marked by unconsciousness and exaggerated reflexes.
    a. Stage 1
    b. Stage 2
    c. Stage 3
    d. Stage 4

14. _____ includes minimal, moderate, and deep sedation.
    a. Dissociative anesthesia
    b. Regional anesthesia
    c. Conscious sedation
    d. Nonreceptive sedation

15. _____ is induced with the drug ketamine.
    a. Dissociative anesthesia
    b. Regional anesthesia
    c. Conscious sedation
    d. Nonreceptive sedation

16. _____ provides reversible loss of sensation in a specific area of the body without affecting consciousness.
    a. Dissociative anesthesia
    b. Regional anesthesia
    c. Conscious sedation
    d. Nonreceptive sedation

17. MAC stands for:
    a. Monitored anesthesia consciousness
    b. Monitored anesthetic care
    c. Monitored anesthesia care
    d. None of the above

18. A _____ anesthetic is an injection into superficial tissue to produce a small area of anesthesia.
    a. Topical
    b. Local
    c. Spinal
    d. Nerve

19. A _____ anesthetic provides anesthesia to a specific area of the body supplied by a major nerve or nerve plexus.
    a. Topical
    b. Local
    c. Spinal
    d. Nerve

20. A _____ anesthetic is used on mucous membranes and on superficial eye tissue during ophthalmic surgery.
    a. Topical
    b. Local
    c. Spinal
    d. Nerve

21. A(n) _____ is injection of anesthetic into the intrathecal space.
    a. Intravenous block
    b. Nerve block
    c. Epidural
    d. Spinal block

22. A _____ is a also known as Bier block.
    a. Intravenous Block
    b. Nerve
    c. Epidural
    d. Spinal

23. A _____ is produced when the anesthetic agent is injected into the epidural space.
    a. Intravenous block
    b. Nerve block
    c. Epidural
    d. Spinal block

24. When the body is in a balanced physiological state, it is in _____
    a. Hemostasis
    b. Balanced anesthesia
    c. Homeostasis
    d. Topical anesthesia

25. Deep unconsciousness, such as that achieved during general anesthesia, results in the absence of protective mechanisms, such as _____.
    a. Blinking and shivering
    b. Cessation of brain activity
    c. Loss of recall
    d. Diminished mental and physical capacity

26. Which of the following is *not* an example of autonomic responses?
    a. Changes in heartbeats
    b. Release of insulin
    c. Peristalsis
    d. Digestion

27. The _____ is responsible for management of postoperative pain.
    a. Surgeon
    b. ACP
    c. RN
    d. Anesthesia tech

28. Hospitals have individual check-in protocols, which may include all of the following details, *except*:
    a. Patient identity
    b. Correct surgical site
    c. Consent forms
    d. Religious preference

29. Which of the following is *not* considered part of the preoperative routine?
    a. Preoperative fasting
    b. Sedative medication
    c. Prophylactic antibiotics
    d. Inhalation agents

30. Which of the following is a purpose of preoperative medication?
    a. Increase anxiety
    b. Begin induction
    c. Increase gastric volume
    d. Reduce the amount of general anesthetic used

31. Which of the following describes physiologic monitoring in the operating room?
    a. A preoperative assessment of the patient's vital metabolic functions
    b. Monitoring that requires patient assessment for clinical signs, interpretation of these signs, and initiation of the appropriate medical response
    c. Physiological monitoring must be done by the anesthesiologist.
    d. Monitoring is necessary because the trauma of surgery has no effect on normal body functions.

32. Which of the following is *not* considered protective reflexes?
    a. Heartbeat
    b. Gagging
    c. Swallowing
    d. Withdrawal from pain

33. Electrocardiography (ECG) measures the:
    a. Heart rate per minute
    b. Electrical activity of the brain
    c. Electrical activity of the heart
    d. Respiratory rate per minute

34. Normal body temperature is _____.
    a. 36° to 37.5° C
    b. 95° to 97° C
    c. 94° to 96° F
    d. 36° to 37.5° F

35. A peripheral nerve block:
    a. Provides anesthesia to a specific area of the body
    b. Involves injection of the anesthetic agent into the nerve
    c. Is enervated by a specific nerve
    d. Is done at the end of the procedure for postoperative pain

36. Which of the following would *not* be needed for a Bier block procedure?
    a. Single bladder tourniquet
    b. Esmarch bandage
    c. IV
    d. Lidocaine

CASE STUDIES

1. *Read the following case study and answer the questions based on your knowledge of the regional drug toxicity and allergic response.*

   Ms. Jones is having surgery. She states that the last time she had surgery, she did not wake up quickly and she was throwing up, had a headache, fast heart-beat, and skin irritation.

   a. What types of reactions was Ms. Jones exhibiting and why?

   b. How do you approach giving Ms. Jones anesthesia for this surgery?

   c. What can the CST monitor during surgery to help ensure Ms. Jones does not have the same issue?

2. *The American Society of Anesthesiologists (ASA) has developed an assessment system that classifies patients according to risk for anesthesia-related complications. Using that information, rate the following patients:*

   a. Your 81-year-old patient comes to the emergency department for acute cholecystitis.

      He is classified as a _____.

   b. Your 18-year-old patient comes to the hospital for an EGD. The patient currently has medically controlled asthma and has had the problem for about 10 years. He is

      mildly obese. He is classified as a _____.

   c. Your 26-year-old patient has come to the hospital for a scheduled cesarean section for delivery of healthy twin babies. She has no underlying disease and will be

      classified as a _____.

   d. Your patient is a 39-year-old woman who has insulin-dependent diabetes. She is completely controlled and has kept her blood glucose within normal range by diet, exercise, and insulin for about 6 years. She is coming to the hospital for a tubal

      ligation. She will be classified as a _____.

Student's Name: _____ Date: _____

Task: Student verbalizes purpose of cricoid pressure.

Equipment and Supplies:

- No equipment required

Evaluation Directions: Check or circle the appropriate number to indicate the student's performance level, using the following rating scale:

3-PROFICIENT. Can complete the task quickly and accurately without direction.

2-PARTIALLY PROFICIENT. Can do most of the task. Needs assistance. Needs constant supervision.

1-LIMITED. Can do a limited amount of the task. Must be told what to do. Needs extremely close supervision.

0-UNSATISFACTORY. Can do a limited amount of the task. Must be told what to do. Needs extremely close supervision.

Task Checklist	Rating	Self-Assessment	Instructor Assessment
1. Position self properly	0 1 2 3		
2. Identify relevant anatomy	0 1 2 3		
3. Position hand properly	0 1 2 3		
4. Apply adequate pressure	0 1 2 3		
5. Maintain cricoid pressure until asked to release	0 1 2 3		
Total Score			

SCORE

15-12 = A

11-9 = B

8-6 = C

Below 6 = not passing

Comments:

_____

_____

_____

_____

15 Postanesthesia Recovery

Student's Name _____

KEY TERMS

Write the definition for each term.

1. Activities of daily living (ADLs) _____

2. Arterial blood gases (ABGs) _____

3. Aspiration _____

4. Auscultation _____

5. Bronchospasm _____

6. Discharge against medical advice _____

7. Discharge criteria _____

8. Glasgow Coma Scale _____

9. Handover (hand off) _____

10. Hypothermia _____

11. Hypoxia _____

12. Laryngospasm _____

13. Malignant hyperthermia (MH) _____

14. Perfusion _____

15. Prognosis _____

SHORT ANSWERS

Provide a short answer for each question or statement.

1. Explain the process when admitting a patient to PACU.

   _____

   _____

2. List the verbal and written information provided in a handover.

_____

_____

3. Why does the perioperative nurse need to report blood loss to the PACU?

_____

_____

4. During a focused patient assessment in PACU, which specific patient criteria are assessed?

_____

_____

5. What is the Glasgow Coma Scale (GSC), and how is it used in the PACU?

_____

_____

6. What areas are assessed with the Glasgow Coma Scale?

_____

_____

7. Discharge planning and implementation follow established roles and tasks. List them.

_____

_____

CASE STUDIES

1. *Read the following case study and follow the instructions based on your knowledge of the PACU.*

   You are talking to a friend who is considering a surgical procedure. She asks you about the recovery unit, and you proceed to tell her how the room is arranged. She asks if you could draw a picture for her. Using your text as a guide, draw in the specific details of the PACU.

2. *You are working in the PACU today. Your patient is an 81-year-old man who has insulin-dependent diabetes mellitus (IDDM) and has just undergone a laparoscopic cholecystectomy for cholelithiasis. You have been asked to see whether he meets the discharge criteria by asking him questions and charting his responses. Each criterion is listed on the following chart. Formulate a question that is appropriate for your PACU patient and then assess whether his response meets the criterion.*

   - *You may need to consult your text to review the criteria.*

   - *Do not forget to use good communication skills for questioning patients. You may need to refer to your text and to Chapter 2 for communication skills.*

Discharge criteria	Question	Have criteria been met?
N&V		
Urinary		
Incision site		
Pain control		
Discharge orders		
Escort		
Home environment		

16 Death and Dying

Student's Name _____

Write the definition for each term.

1. Advance health care directive: _____

2. Coroner's case: _____

3. Cultural competence: _____

4. Determination of death: _____

5. DNAR: _____

6. DNR: _____

7. End of life: _____

8. Heart beating cadaver: _____

9. Kübler-Ross, Elisabeth: _____

10. Living will: _____

11. Non–heart beating cadaver: _____

12. Postmortem care: _____

13. Required request law: _____

14. Rigor mortis: _____

SHORT ANSWER

Provide a short answer for each question or statement.

1. From a medical point of view, the *end of life* is:

   _____

   _____

2. The term *brain dead* refers to:

_____

_____

3. _____ is the right of every individual to make decisions about how he or she lives and dies.

4. _____ issues arise when decisions about end-of-life care fall to the family when the patient is unable to communicate his or her wishes.

5. _____ or _____ expresses the patient decision to decline lifesaving efforts.

6. _____ care is the medical and supportive care provided to the dying patient.

7. Describe briefly the difference between a living will and a DNR order.

_____

_____

MATCHING

Match the term with the description.

1. _____ It may occur during the dying process, but treated clinically.

2. _____ A natural first response, a defense mechanism.

3. _____ The idea that death is no longer a source of psychological conflict.

4. _____ Refusing nutrition or treatment.

5. _____ "I just want to experience one pain-free day with my family."

a. Denial
b. Bargaining
c. Anger
d. Acceptance
e. Depression

MULTIPLE CHOICE

Choose the most correct answer to complete the question or statement.

1. Which of the following is a famous physiatrist who constructed the death and dying model that is most frequently recognized today?
   a. Maslow
   b. Freud
   c. Piaget
   d. Elisabeth Kübler-Ross

2. During the dying process, _____ is a defense mechanism that forestalls the full impact of the fact of death until the mind is ready to accept it.
   a. Denial
   b. Acceptance
   c. Bargaining
   d. Anger

3. A dying patient may express anger to:
   a. Gain control over the environment
   b. Get even with the physician
   c. Pass through the stages of dying even if the person is not angry
   d. Keep from becoming depressed

4. It is the responsibility of the _____ to convey information about the patient's medical condition to the family and/or friends.
   a. Operating room scheduler or secretary
   b. Surgeon only
   c. Medical and nursing staff
   d. Operating room staff

5. The order to _____ is made official by signing a DNR order, which is charted in the patient's medical record.
   a. Not resuscitate
   b. Call the doctor
   c. Add additional medications
   d. Sign a surgical consent form

6. Examples of palliative care include all of the following, *except:*
   a. Debulking of a tumor
   b. X-ray films
   c. DeBakey debridement of a pressure wound
   d. Insertion of a gastric feeding tube

7. When a surgical technologist is providing information to family or friends about a patient's medical condition, it is appropriate for the technologist only to:
   a. Report that the surgery is taking longer than usual
   b. Report that the patient is in good hands and is doing well
   c. Offer an acknowledgment of loss
   d. Discuss the laboratory test values

8. The surgical technologist should refrain from providing information to family or friends about _____ of the patient.
   a. A financial report
   b. Counseling
   c. The mental status
   d. The medical condition

9. For surgical technologists to recognize and acknowledge the fact of death and what this means to the patient in that moment and time, they should:
   a. Focus on what the patient is experiencing in the operating room or holding area.
   b. Observe facial expressions and gestures
   c. Be alert to any changes in mood or signs of anxiety and fear related to death and isolation
   d. All of the above

10. Medical interventions for a dying patient include all of the following, *except:*
    a. Respiratory support (artificial respiration)
    b. Intravenous feeding
    c. Dialysis
    d. Pain medications

11. The _____ of death is considered by some to be too constricting and does not allow for individualism in the experience of death.
    a. Stage theory
    b. End of life theory
    c. Spiritual theory
    d. Psychological theory
    e. Examination

12. _____ is the right of every individual to make decisions about how he or she lives and dies.
    a. DNR
    b. Advance directive
    c. Self-determination
    d. Living will

13. A _____ specifies the exact nature of palliative care that a patient accepts.
    a. Living will
    b. Advance directive
    c. DNR
    d. Assisted suicide

14. When no verifiable permission has been granted for organ donation by the patient, the _____ may act as a surrogate for the patient.
    a. Surgeon
    b. Family
    c. Chaplain
    d. Nurses

15. In the operating room, death is a(n) _____ event.
    a. Rare
    b. Occasional
    c. Weekly
    d. Daily

16. For a coroner's case, all of the following are mandatory for an autopsy, *except:*
    a. Death of an incarcerated individual
    b. Unwitnessed death
    c. Death after admission from the same facility
    d. Suicide

17. Donors are registered in different _____ of the country and the data are exchanged with recovery organizations.
    a. Parts
    b. States
    c. Regions
    d. Counties

18. Reactions and coping skills available to health care professionals are influenced by the following factors, *except:*
    a. Lack of support
    b. The health care professional's beliefs and values
    c. Previous experience with death
    d. Emotional well-being

19. A _____ cadaver is maintained on cardiopulmonary support to provide tissue perfusion.
    a. Non-heart-beating
    b. Heart-beating

20. A _____ cadaver is restricted to those who do not need perfusion to sustain viability for later transplantation.
   a. Non–heart-beating
   b. Heart-beating

21. Organ and tissue donation arises as a(n) _____ issue when the patient has not left a clear directive before death.
   a. Moral
   b. Ethical

22. _____ prepares the body for viewing by the family and assists in further handling procedures carried out by the morgue and mortuary.
   a. Rigor mortis
   b. Operating room
   c. Postmortem care
   d. All the above

23. The process of recovery is administered through:
   a. Donors
   b. Tissue banks
   c. Recipients
   d. Organized recovery
   e. All the above

CASE STUDIES

1. *Read the following case study and answer the questions based on your knowledge of death and dying.*

   You are called in for an exploratory laparotomy. Upon arrival to the hospital, you learn your patient has a ruptured aneurysm. You prepare the operating room and scrub, then notice the patient is brought in and is not breathing. The surgeon makes the incision and the abdomen is filled with blood and your patient crashes. After a very brief silence, you patient dies on the table.

   a. What is your role as a surgical technologist at this point?

   b. You are called upstairs to do an emergency C-section. What is your role?

   c. The patient's family wants to see their family member. Who stays with the family while they say good bye?

d. What is the ethical thing to do with this patient?

e. Do you remove all the cords, clean the patient up before the family visit? Why?

17 Physics and Information Technology

Student's Name _____

 1. Alternating current (AC): _____

 2. Ampere: _____

 3. Amplitude: _____

 4. Atom: _____

 5. Boiling point: _____

 6. Central processing unit (CPU): _____

 7. Circuit: _____

 8. Coherent light waves: _____

 9. Conduction: _____

10. Conductivity: _____

11. Convection: _____

12. Database: _____

13. Direct current (DC): _____

14. Doppler effect: _____

15. Doppler ultrasound: _____

16. Electromagnetic field: _____

17. Electromagnetic waves: _____

18. Electron: _____

19. Electrostatic discharge: _____

20. Element: _____

21. Focal point: _____

22. Frequency: _____

23. Gravitational energy: _____

24. Harmonics: _____

25. Hot wire: _____

26. Hyperlinks: _____

27. Insulator: _____

28. Internal drives: _____

29. Internet: _____

30. Intranet: _____

31. Isotope: _____

32. Kinetic energy: _____

33. Magnetic field: _____

34. Molecule: _____

35. Momentum: _____

36. Neutron: _____

37. Nucleus: _____

38. Periodic table: _____

39. Photon: _____

40. Plasma: _____

41. Potential energy: _____

42. Receptacle: _____

43. Reflection: _____

44. Refraction: _____

45. Resistance: _____

46. Serial lenses: _____

47. Solid: _____

48. States of matter: _____

49. Static electricity: _____

50. Thermal conductivity: _____

51. Thermoregulation: _____

52. Ultrasound: _____

53. Voltage: _____

54. Wave: _____

55. Wavelength: _____

56. World Wide Web: _____

SHORT ANSWERS

Provide a short answer for each question or statement.

1. List the five areas of study in mechanics and physics, and define.

   a. _____

   b. _____

   c. _____

   d. _____

   e. _____

2. What are the four states of matter? Give an example of each.

   a. _____

   b. _____

   c. _____

   d. _____

3. What are the five elements of motion? Give an example of each.

   a. _____

   b. _____

   c. _____

   d. _____

   e. _____

4. List the five types of energy, define, and give an example of each.

   a. _____

   b. _____

   c. _____

   d. _____

   e. _____

Chapter **17 Physics and Information Technology**

MATCHING

Match each term with the correct definition as it applies to heat.

1. _____ The term for different substances having differing abilities to conduct or transmit heat.

2. _____ Creates a current as the warm air rises and cool air falls

3. _____ The ability of a substance to conduct heat.

4. _____ The transfer of heat by electromagnetic waves.

5. _____ The displacement of cool air by warm air.

6. _____ A complex physiological process in which the body maintains a temperature that is optimal for survival.

7. _____ The transfer of heat from one substance to another by the natural movement of molecules, which sets other molecules in motion.

a. Conduction

b. Convection

c. Radiation

d. Thermal conductivity

e. Thermoregulation

MATCHING

Match each term with the correct definition as it applies to matter.

1. _____ A pure substance composed of atoms, each with the same number of protons.

2. _____ A positively charged subatomic particle that is part of the nucleus of an atom.

3. _____One of the three states or properties of a substance in which the temperature reached the melting point.

4. _____ A state of matter in which the molecules are bonded very tightly.

5. _____ A discrete unit made of matter consisting of charged particles.

6. _____ A charge particle created when an atom loses or gains an electron.

7. _____ An atom of a specific element with the correct number of electrons and protons but a different number of neutrons.

8. _____ A specific substance made up of elements that are bonded together.

9. _____ A subatomic particle located in the nucleus of the atom that has no electrical charge.

10. _____ A negatively charged particle that orbits the nucleus of an atom.

a. Atom

b. Isotope

c. Molecule

d. Electron

e. Neutron

f. Element

g. Ion

h. Proton

i. Solid

j. Liquids

MATCHING

Match the term with the definition.

1. _____ Memory
2. _____ Motherboard
3. _____ Drive
4. _____ Monitor
5. _____ Keyboard
6. _____ Mouse
7. _____ Speakers
8. _____ Hard copy

a. Alphanumeric device for inputting data into the computer
b. Also called RAM
c. Data from computer which has been reproduced in the form of a CD
d. The computer screen where data is viewed by the user
e. Provides sound output from the computer
f. The primary circuits that run the computer
g. The user's steering component
h. Internal or external device that stores the computer's data

MULTIPLE CHOICE

Choose the most correct answer to complete the question or statement.

1. Free electrons flow through conductive material in a continuous path, each electron "pushing" the one ahead of it. This is called a(n) _____.
   a. Circuit
   b. Static electricity
   c. Polarity
   d. Alternating current

2. "The natural attractive force of masses in the universe" defines:
   a. Gravitational energy
   b. Kinetic energy
   c. Chemical energy
   d. Nuclear energy

3. Which of the following is smallest?
   a. Electron
   b. Proton
   c. Neutron
   d. Atomic nucleus

4. The atomic number of an element corresponds to the element's:
   a. Number of electrons
   b. Number of protons
   c. Number of neutrons
   d. Placement on the periodic table

5. Organic compounds all have molecules that contain the element _____.
   a. Iron
   b. Hydrogen
   c. Carbon
   d. Ions

6. "Mass $\times$ velocity" is the equation for:
   a. Force
   b. Momentum
   c. Distance
   d. Propulsion

7. The distance around a circle is called the
   _____.
   a. Force
   b. Momentum
   c. Circumference
   d. Projectile motion

8. Potential energy is also referred to as
   _____.
   a. Energy potential
   b. Electrical energy
   c. Mechanical energy
   d. Stored energy

9. The _____ protects the circuit from a "short" or fault in the system.
   a. Active wire
   b. Neutral wire
   c. Ground wire
   d. Electrical circuit

10. When light rays encounter some surfaces, they can reverse direction; this is called:
    a. Refractive index
    b. Refraction
    c. Reflection
    d. Coherence

11. _____ is when a wave reaches a boundary.
    a. Reflection
    b. Wavelength
    c. Amplitude
    d. Frequency

12. _____ is the point of greatest disturbance.
    a. Reflection
    b. Wavelength
    c. Amplitude
    d. Frequency

13. _____ is the measurement of one complete wave cycle.
    a. Reflection
    b. Wavelength
    c. Amplitude
    d. Frequency

14. _____ is the number of waves that pass a point in 1 second.
    a. Reflection
    b. Wavelength
    c. Amplitude
    d. Frequency

15. A(n) _____ program performs the functions of a typewriter with many additional features.
    a. Word processing
    b. Database
    c. Graphic design
    d. Interactive education

16. A(n) _____ type of program allows the user to enter complex data involving items, lists, and numerical or arithmetic information.
    a. Word processing
    b. Database
    c. Graphic design
    d. Interactive education

17. A(n) _____ type of program provides the computing tools needed to "draw" and manipulate figures or to create complex images based on quantitative data.
    a. Word processing
    b. Database
    c. Graphic design
    d. Interactive education

18. _____ programs are designed to help the user learn subjects such as mathematics, languages, and physical sciences.
    a. Word processing
    b. Database
    c. Graphic design
    d. Interactive education

19. This is known as the:

    a. Desktop
    b. Window
    c. Toolbar
    d. Menu

20. This is known as the:

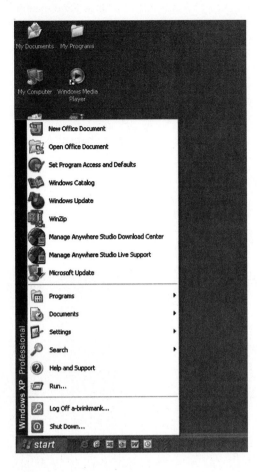

a. CPU
b. Window
c. Toolbar
d. Menu

21. This is known as the:

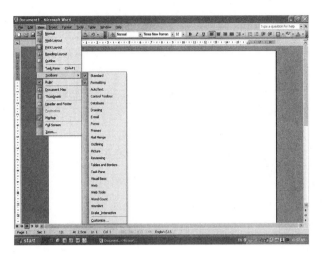

a. CPU
b. Window
c. Toolbar
d. Menu

CASE STUDIES

1. *Read the following case study and answer the questions based on your knowledge of motion.*

   Today you are at the park studying for your examination on energy and motion. You notice the children in the park, who are all playing on the toys there. Describe each type of energy or motion exhibited by each of the following children.

   a. Tom and Sally are playing on a teeter-totter.

      The motion they are exhibiting is _____.

      They energy they are exhibiting is _____.

   b. Jon is playing on a swing set. He is swinging alone.

      The motion that Jon is exhibiting is _____.

      The movement is called _____.

c. Karen and Emily are playing on the merry-go-round.

The motion that they are exhibiting is _____.

d. Jacob is dropping sticks off the bridge into the water. What type of energy is Jacob exhibiting? _____

18 Energy Sources in Surgery

Student's Name _____

Write the definition for each term.

1. Ablation: _____

2. Active electrode: _____

3. Active electrode monitoring (AEM): _____

4. Alternating current (AC): _____

5. Amplification: _____

6. Argon: _____

7. Bipolar circuit: _____

8. Blended mode: _____

9. Capacitive coupling: _____

10. Carbon dioxide: _____

11. Cauterization: _____

12. Cavitron ultrasonic surgical aspirator (CUSA): _____

13. Circuit: _____

14. Coagulum: _____

15. Coherency: _____

16. Conductive: _____

17. Continuous wave lasers: _____

18. Cryoablation: _____

19. Cryosurgery: _____

20. Current: _____

21. Cavitron ultrasonic surgical aspirator (CUSA): _____

22. Cutting mode: _____

23. Desiccation: _____

24. Direct coupling: _____

25. Direct current (DC): _____

26. Dispersive electrode: _____

27. Duty cycle: _____

28. Electrosurgery: _____

29. Electrosurgical unit (ESU): _____

30. Electrosurgical vessel sealing: _____

31. Electrosurgical waveforms: _____

32. Eschar: _____

33. Excimer: _____

34. Excitation source: _____

35. Frequency: _____

36. Fulguration: _____

37. Grounding pad: _____

38. Holmium:YAG: _____

39. Impedance: _____

40. Implanted electronic device (IED): _____

41. Inactive electrode: _____

42. Insulate: _____

43. Isolated circuit: _____

44. Laser: _____

45. Laser classifications: _____

46. Laser head: _____

47. Laser medium: _____

48. Lateral heat: _____

49. Monochromatic: _____

50. Monopolar circuit: _____

51. Neodymium:YAG: _____

52. Neutral electrode: _____

53. Nonconductive: _____

54. Optical resonant cavity: _____

55. Patient return electrode (PRE): _____

56. Phacoemulsification: _____

57. Potassium-titanyl-phosphate (KTP): _____

58. Pulsed wave lasers: _____

59. Q-switched lasers: _____

60. Radiant exposure: _____

61. Radiofrequency: _____

62. Radiofrequency ablation (RFA): _____

63. Resistance: _____

64. Return electrode monitoring (REM): _____

65. Selective absorption: _____

66. Smoke plume: _____

67. Spray coagulation: _____

68. Tunable dye laser: _____

69. Ultrasonic energy: _____

In monopolar electrosurgery, the electrical current passes into the patient's body and makes a complete circuit or a circular path. Label the picture by using the numbers provided.

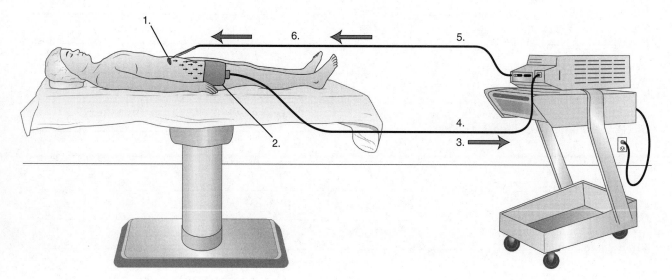

1.

2.

3.

4.

5.

6.

LABELING

Name the bovie tip and description of use.

1.

2.

3.

4.

5.

6.

7.

8.

9.

10.

11.

12.

13.

14.

15.

16.

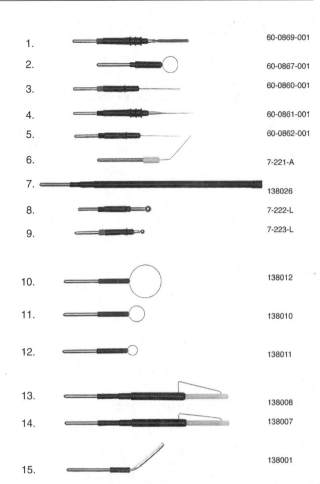

1.	60-0869-001
2.	60-0867-001
3.	60-0860-001
4.	60-0861-001
5.	60-0862-001
6.	7-221-A
7.	138026
8.	7-222-L
9.	7-223-L
10.	138012
11.	138010
12.	138011
13.	138008
14.	138007
15.	138001
16.	138000

Courtesy Conmed, Inc.

SHORT ANSWERS

Provide a short answer for each question or statement.

1. Which variables cause tissue to react to electrosurgery?

2. Describe the difference between cautery, electrosurgery, and ultrasound.

3. What is the difference between monopolar and bipolar delivery of ESU?

_____

_____

4. What is capacitive coupling and why would it occur in endoscopic procedures more often than in open procedures?

_____

_____

5. How do lasers work?

_____

_____

6. How are lasers classified?

_____

_____

7. Lasers are grouped into two categories according to the duration of the output waves. What are the two groups?

a.

b.

Student's Name _____

KEY TERMS

Write the definition for each term.

1. Abduction: _____

2. Compartment syndrome: _____

3. Compression injury: _____

4. Dependent area of the body: _____

5. Embolism: _____

6. Fasciotomy: _____

7. Foot board: _____

8. Hyperextension: _____

9. Hyperflexion: _____

10. Hypotension: _____

11. Ischemia: _____

12. Lateral transfer: _____

13. Necrosis: _____

14. Neuropathy: _____

15. Range of motion: _____

16. Shear injury: _____

17. Thoracic outlet syndrome: _____

18. Thromboembolus (embolus): _____

19. Traction injury: _____

20. Transfer board: _____

21. Trendelenburg position: _____

LABELING

Label the operating room table in the following figure.

1.

2.

3.

4.

5.

6.

7.

8.

9.

10.

11.

Modified from Martin JT, Warner MA: *Positioning in anesthesia and surgery*, ed 3, Philadelphia, 1997, WB Saunders.

SHORT ANSWERS

Provide a short answer for each question or statement.

1. How and why is a transfer board used?

_____

_____

2. What type of activity would or could cause a shearing injury?

_____

_____

3. Why are health care workers at high risk for back injury and musculoskeletal injury while moving and transferring patients?

_____

_____

4. List three risk factors for patient injury when patients are transported or transferred:

   a.

   b.

   c.

5. What are the three ways that all health care workers should identify the patient?

   a.

   b.

   c.

6. What are the steps taken to transfer a patient from a bed to a wheelchair?

   _____

   _____

7. What are the steps taken to assist a patient in moving from a lying position to a sitting position?

   _____

   _____

8. Name the three elements of safe positioning of a patient.

   a.

   b.

   c.

9. List the injuries that occur during transport and transfer.

   _____

   _____

10. List the principles that apply to all types of patient transport and transfer.

    _____

    _____

Match each term with the correct definition. Some terms may be used more than once.

1. _D_ Position in which the patient's head is tilted down
2. _e_ Position in which the patient is lying on the back
3. _h_ Sitting position
4. _a_ Position in which the patient's feet are tilted down
5. _b_ Position in which the patient is lying with the front of the body (the abdomen) on the operating room table
6. _c_ Position used for vaginal, perineal, and rectal procedures
7. _e_ Position used for neck and thyroid procedures
8. _f_ A type of prone position in which the patient's hips are flexed in an inverted V
9. _h_ Sitting position used for cranial, facial, and reconstructive breast procedures
10. _g_ Side-lying position
11. _b_ Position used for spine, cranium, and perianal procedures

a. Reverse Trendelenburg position
b. Prone position
c. Lithotomy position
d. Trendelenburg position
e. Supine position
f. Jackknife (Kraske) position
g. Lateral position
h. Fowler position

MATCHING

Match the pressure ulcer stage with the correct term.

1. _____ Partial-thickness skin loss involving the epidermis and/or dermis. A superficial ulcer evolves and develops clinically as an abrasion, a blister, or a shallow crater.

2. _____ Full-thickness skin loss with extensive destruction, tissue necrosis, or damage to muscle, bone, or supporting structures

3. _____ Nonblanchable erythema of intact skin, the heralding lesion of skin ulceration.

4. _____ Full-thickness skin loss, involving damage to or necrosis of subcutaneous tissue that may extend down to but not through underlying fascia. The ulcer presents clinically as a deep crater with or without undermining of adjacent tissue.

a. Stage I
b. Stage II
c. Stage III
d. Stage IV

MULTIPLE CHOICE

Choose the most correct answer to complete the question or statement.

1. Which of the following terms means movement of a joint or body part away from the body?
   a. Abduction
   b. Adduction
   c. Hyperextension
   d. Ischemia

2. Health care workers are at high risk for injury while caring for, moving, and transferring patients because:
   a. They do not use proper body mechanics when moving a patient.
   b. The tasks are unpredictable.
   c. A sudden shift of the patient's weight may put the worker off balance.
   d. All of the above.

3. Transport and transfer injuries occur more often when:
   a. There is sufficient help.
   b. Personnel assisting in the transfer or transport have a plan.
   c. Personnel are rushed.
   d. The patient is cooperative.

4. Which of the following statements is true regarding patient transfers?
   a. One person should be in charge of the move and guide the others.
   b. It is best to make a plan as you move the patient so that the move is individualized.
   c. The patient's right to modesty is forfeited at admission.
   d. It is best to move the patient without blankets so that the patient does not get tangled up in them.

5. The most important part of transporting patients is:
   a. Proper identification before you transport them
   b. Proper positioning on the cart
   c. Keeping the patient warm while in the hallways
   d. Greeting the patient in a friendly manner and introducing yourself

6. The first step in transferring a mobile patient to a stretcher is to:
   a. Lower the bed rails and align the patient's bed and the stretcher
   b. Make sure the locks are engaged on both the patient's bed and the stretcher
   c. Identify the patient
   d. Let the surgeon know that the patient is about to be transferred

7. _____ people should be present during the transfer of a mobile and alert patient.
   a. Two or three
   b. Three or four
   c. Four or five
   d. Five or six

8. The transfer of a conscious patient from a stretcher to an operating table starts with aligning the head of the stretcher with the head of the operating table and then:
   a. Opening up the back of the patient's gown
   b. Identifying the patient
   c. Freeing up the IV tubing
   d. Locking the wheels of the stretcher and the operating room table

9. During the transfer of a conscious patient to the operating room table, the duties of the anesthesiologist include:
   a. Protecting the patient's neck and airway
   b. Holding the IV tubing
   c. Controlling the slide board
   d. Nothing; the anesthesiologist does not assist in the move

10. Position a morbidly obese patient on a _____ surgical table.
    a. Standard
    b. Double
    c. Jackson frame
    d. Bariatric

1. *Read the following case study and answer the questions based on your knowledge of patient positioning and use of the operating room table.*

   You have been asked to set up the operating room for a procedure. Today your surgeon will perform an open thoracotomy in operating room 2. The surgeon has told the team that he will be making an incision in the right intercostal area.

   a. In what position will the patient be placed?

   b. What position will the patient be in for administration of the general anesthetic?

   c. What positioning devices will be needed for this patient?

2. *Read the following case study and answer the questions based on your knowledge of patient transfer.*

   You are the assistant circulator in Room 16. The circulator is bringing the patient back to the OR when she calls for extra moving help. You return to the room and notice the patient is obese.

   a. What type of OR table should you have?

b. How many people should help transfer this patient?

c. What types of devices should you have available to assist in the transfer?

d. What type of tissue damage should you be looking for?

3. *Read the following case study and answer the questions based on your knowledge of the pregnant patient.*

You are called in for an emergency appendectomy. You are told upon arrival that your patient is pregnant.

a. What position will the patient be placed in?

b. What position devices should you have available?

c. What type of transfer devices should you have available?

d. What anatomy should you be aware of when positioning this patient?

20 Surgical Skin Prep and Draping

Student's Name _____

KEY TERMS

Write the definition for each term.

1. Antiseptic: _____

2. Debridement: _____

3. Fenestrated drape: _____

4. Impervious: _____

5. Incise drape: _____

6. Residual activity: _____

7. Retention catheter: _____

8. Single-stage prep: _____

9. Solution: _____

10. Straight catheter: _____

11. Surgical site infection (SSI): _____

12. Tincture: _____

In the drawings below, use a colored pen or pencil to indicate the prep for the procedure listed.

1. Anterior head and neck

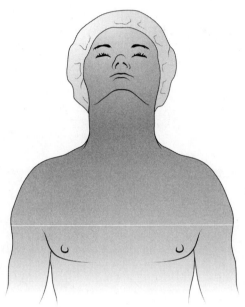

Modified from Phillips N: *Berry and Kohn's operating room technique*, ed 10, St Louis, 2004, Mosby.

2. Anterior shoulder

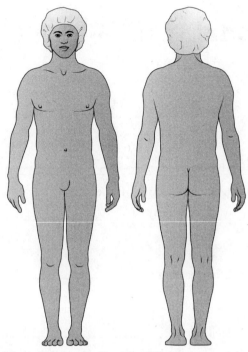

Modified from Phillips N: *Berry and Kohn's operating room technique*, ed 10, St Louis, 2004, Mosby.

3. Back

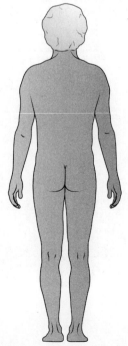

Modified from Phillips N: *Berry and Kohn's operating room technique*, ed 10, St Louis, 2004, Mosby.

4. Abdomen

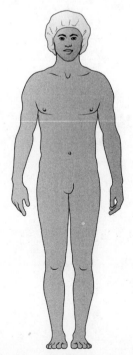

Modified from Phillips N: *Berry and Kohn's operating room technique*, ed 10, St Louis, 2004, Mosby.

Chapter **20 Surgical Skin Prep and Draping**

5. Inguinal area

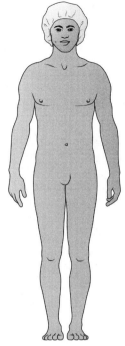

Modified from Phillips N: *Berry and Kohn's operating room technique*, ed 10, St Louis, 2004, Mosby.

SHORT ANSWERS

Provide a short answer for each question or statement.

1. What is the protocol for patient hygiene before surgery? Why is it important?

   _____

   _____

2. List the supplies needed for urinary catheterization.

   _____

   _____

3. List the steps of urinary catheterization.

   _____

   _____

4. List the two types of catheterizations and define. List the types of catheters necessary to perform these types of catheterizations.

_____

_____

5. Urinary catheterization is necessary in selected procedures and circumstances. What are they?

_____

_____

6. What are the risks involved in improper use of prep solutions?

_____

_____

7. Why is iodine a risk of thermal burn when it is heated (warmed)?

_____

_____

8. What measures are taken to ensure that the correct site is prepped?

_____

_____

9. What guidelines should be followed for hair clipping?

_____

_____

10. The flank and back areas are prepped in the same manner as the abdomen; describe the technique.

_____

_____

11. What is the purpose of surgical draping?

_____

_____

12. Before starting the skin prep, the surgical technologist should perform a mental check of patient safety considerations. This includes:

_____

_____

13. List the technique on how to drape equipment.

_____

_____

14. List the technique in draping.

_____

_____

15. List the technique in removing drapes.

_____

_____

MATCHING

Match each term with the correct definition. Some terms may be used more than once.

1. ___C___ destroys microorganisms by *desiccation* (drying) of the cell proteins.

2. ___f___ has not been approved as a first-choice skin prep by The Joint Commission or CDC.

3. ___b___ is absorbed through the skin and may cause toxicity. Although it normally is nonirritating to tissue, first-degree and second-degree chemical burns can result from improper prep technique or if the patient is sensitive to iodine.

4. ___d___ an antiseptic commonly found in deodorants, antibacterial soaps, and other proprietary cosmetics.

5. ___e___ is labeled for use around the eye, mouth, or genital area, especially as an alternative to povidone-iodine.

6. ___a___ The FDA's most recent decision on prep solution is that the antiseptic is not generally recognized as safe and effective for use as an antiseptic hand wash and should not be used to bathe patients with burns or extensive areas of susceptible, sensitive skin.

a. Hexachlorophene
b. Iodophors
c. Alcohol
d. Triclosan
e. Parachlorometaxylenol
f. Chlorhexidine gluconate (CHG)

Choose the most correct answer to complete the question or statement.

1. Uncontrolled or unmonitored systems create a risk of:
   a. Allergies
   b. Chemical burn
   c. Fire
   d. Thermal burn

2. Surgical prep agents can cause skin irritation, rash, or other:
   a. Reactions
   b. Chemical burn
   c. Fire
   d. Thermal burn

3. Alcohol and alcohol-based prep solutions are volatile and flammable. When alcohol solution or volatile fumes come in contact with heat sources, they can easily cause:
   a. Allergies
   b. Chemical burn
   c. Fire
   d. Thermal burn

4. Serious _____ can occur when prep solutions are allowed to pool under the patient during surgery
   a. Allergies
   b. Chemical burns
   c. Fires
   d. Thermal burns

5. During the cleansing process, the surgeon removes all foreign material and trims away devitalized tissue called:
   a. Trauma
   b. Cardiac/vascular
   c. Autograft
   d. Debridement

6. _____ is a type of tissue that is removed from one site on the patient and grafted to another site.
   a. Trauma
   b. Cardiac/vascular
   c. Autograft
   d. Debridement

7. _____ wounds are almost always contaminated because they are caused by external forces and often occur in environments that are mildly or grossly contaminated.
   a. Trauma
   b. Cardiac/vascular
   c. Autograft
   d. Debridement

8. _____ require a large area of exposure.
   a. Trauma wounds
   b. Cardiac/vascular inscisions
   c. Autografts
   d. Debridement

9. _____ are folded in a specific way before sterilization so that they can be positioned over the operative site and unfolded in a way that prevents contamination.
   a. Towels
   b. Gowns
   c. Drapes
   d. All the above

10. The patient is ready for skin prep and draping only after:
    a. Induction of general anesthesia and intubation
    b. The "pause"
    c. The circulator has finished the required surgical paperwork
    d. The surgeon inspects the patient's surgical site skin

11. A retention catheter with a small, inflatable balloon at the tip is called a _____ catheter.
    a. Robinson
    b. Malecot
    c. Fogarty
    d. Foley

12. Selection of the correct catheter is based on the patient's:
    a. Age, mental development, and sexual preference
    b. Age, size, and the type of procedure
    c. Age, size, and gender
    d. Size, grade in school, and gender

13. Catheterization of a female surgical patient requires the _____ position.
    a. Supine
    b. Prone
    c. Lithotomy
    d. Knees slightly flexed

14. Which of the following statements is true regarding the technique for placing a Foley catheter?
    a. The assisting hand does not contact sterile supplies, including the catheter itself.
    b. Both hands must remain sterile for the procedure.
    c. If the catheter is placed before the prep has been done, it is not done using aseptic technique.
    d. The insertion hand does not contact sterile supplies.

15. Healthy skin contains colonies of:
    a. Infection
    b. Bacteria
    c. Grease
    d. Water

16. When is hair removed from the surgical site?
    a. When it is ordered by the surgeon
    b. When it will interfere with the procedure
    c. When the patient has excess hair
    d. When the patient is a high risk for surgical site infection

17. Which of the following is *not* true regarding the two methods of prepping?
    a. Antiseptic soap solution is used, followed by a coating of antiseptic.
    b. Antiseptic solution alone is used.
    c. The prep used is based on the surgeon's orders.
    d. The prep used is based on the preferences of the hospital infection control nurse.

18. The basic principles of the skin prep:
    a. Vary from patient to patient
    b. Are based on the rules of aseptic technique
    c. Vary from procedure to procedure
    d. Are based on hospital policy and surgeon's preference

19. Surgeons apply the surgical drapes in a prescribed order based on:
    a. Aseptic technique
    b. Surgical practice
    c. The patient's risk of infection
    d. Hospital policy

20. To ensure a moisture barrier between the patient and the sterile field, surgical drapes are made of woven and _____ materials.
    a. Polypropylene
    b. Linen
    c. Bonded synthetic
    d. Polyester

21. A draping routine usually begins with:
    a. A plain sheet
    b. A stockinette
    c. A fenestrated drape
    d. A towel or sticky drape

22. The sterile drape that is coated with adhesive on one side and may be impregnated with antiseptic is called a(n):
    a. Three-quarter drape
    b. Fenestrated drape
    c. Half-sheet
    d. Incise drape

23. The procedure drape, or specialty drape, is placed on the patient:
    a. Before the half-sheet
    b. Before the incise drape
    c. First
    d. Last

24. Which of the following rules of asepsis apply to placement of the surgical drapes?
    a. Handle drapes with as much movement as you need to ensure proper placement.
    b. When placing a drape, do not touch the patient's body.
    c. After a drape has been placed, shift or move the drape to make a good fit for the patient and the procedure.
    d. Use towel clamps to secure drapes.

25. The sterile technique required for catheterization entails keeping:
    a. Both hands and arms sterile
    b. Both hands unsterile, because this is not a sterile procedure
    c. One hand sterile and the other hand nonsterile
    d. Both hands sterile

26. _____ is the most common HAI.
    a. Surgical site
    b. Urinary catheterization
    c. Improper prep
    d. All the above

1. *Read the following case study and answer the questions based on your knowledge of insertion of a urinary catheter.*

   Your surgical patient has been released to you for prepping and draping by the anesthesia provider. The surgeon has requested placement of a Foley catheter for this procedure.

   a. Before you begin the procedure, you check the patient's chart for allergies. Why is this particularly important for placement of a Foley catheter?

   b. What is the job of the "assisting hand" during insertion of a urinary catheter?

   c. What is the job of the "insertion hand" during urinary catheter insertion?

2. *Read the following case study and answer the questions based on your knowledge of surgical drapes.*

   You are about to scrub for a knee arthroscopy. Your patient is asleep under general anesthesia. He has been prepped, and you are about to drape him. What will you need to have ready for the surgeon so that you can drape the patient? List your supplies in the order you will use them.

Student's Name:_____ Date: _____

Task: Student demonstrates the ability to perform urinary catheterization.

Equipment and Supplies:

- Sterile gloves
- Catheter supplies

Evaluation Directions: Check or circle the appropriate number to indicate the student's performance level, using the following rating scale:

3-PROFICIENT. Can complete the task quickly and accurately without direction.

2-PARTIALLY PROFICIENT. Can do most of the task. Needs assistance. Needs constant supervision.

1-LIMITED. Can do a limited amount of the task. Must be told what to do. Needs extremely close supervision.

0-UNSATISFACTORY. Can do a limited amount of the task. Must be told what to do. Needs extremely close supervision.

Task Checklist	Rating	Self-Assessment	Instructor Assessment
1. Assemble all equipment and supplies.	0 1 2 3		
2. Wash hands.	0 1 2 3		
3. Position and expose patient.	0 1 2 3		
4. Open catheter kit.	0 1 2 3		
5. Don sterile gloves using proper technique.	0 1 2 3		
6. Organize supplies using sterile technique.	0 1 2 3		
7. Apply sterile drapes that are supplied in the catheterization kit.	0 1 2 3		
8. Cleanse meatus using the proper technique.	0 1 2 3		
9. Lubricate tip of catheter.	0 1 2 3		
10. Invert catheter, and look for urine return.	0 1 2 3		
11. Inflate balloon.	0 1 2 3		
12. Secure catheter to patient's leg, if needed.	0 1 2 3		
13. Wash hands after procedure.	0 1 2 3		
Total Score			

SCORE

39-35 = A

34-30 = B

29-25 = C

24 = not passing

Comments:

_____

_____

_____

_____

21 Case Planning and Intraoperative Routine

Student's Name _____

KEY TERMS

Write the definition for each term.

1. Biopsy: _____

2. Blunt dissection: _____

3. Case planning: _____

4. Count: _____

5. Dissecting sponge: _____

6. Event related: _____

7. Frozen section: _____

8. Graft: _____

9. Implant: _____

10. Radiopaque: _____

11. Raytec: _____

12. Sponge stick: _____

13. Sterile setup: _____

14. Surgeon's preference card: _____

15. TIMEOUT: _____

SHORT ANSWERS

Provide a short answer for each question or statement.

1. What are the four categories of surgical procedures?

   a. _____

   b. _____

   c. _____

   d. _____

2. How will you know what your assignment is and whom your preceptor will be in the operating room on your clinical day?

   _____

   _____

3. What items are typically found on the surgeon's preference card?

   _____

   _____

4. What is a "suture book"?

   _____

   _____

5. What items are included in a surgical count?

   _____

   _____

6. Who is responsible for ensuring that no item is left in a patient?

   _____

   _____

7. When are surgical counts performed?

   _____

   _____

8. Items are usually counted in a specific order; what is that order?

_____

_____

9. What is included in a TIMEOUT?

_____

_____

10. How can a needlestick be prevented in the operating room?

_____

_____

11. Identification of specimens is a critical aspect of surgery. Each specimen must be identified with the following information:

_____

_____

Match each term with the correct description.

1. _____ Means to remove a large portion, but not all of a tumor.

2. _____ Separation of tissue without using sharp instruments.

3. _____ This term means to carefully separate anatomical structures by cutting with instruments, small firm sponges, or the fingers.

4. _____ This term usually refers to the removal of a limb or digit.

5. _____ To constrict by tying

6. _____ This refers to the joining of two hollow anatomical structures (vessels, ducts, tubes, or hollow organs) using sutures or surgical staples.

7. _____ The use of sharp surgical instruments such as a scalpel and scissors to cut away dead tissue

8. _____ To bring a tissue structure partially outside the body.

9. _____ To raise or lift an anatomical structure, sometimes without removing it.

10. _____ is the removal of tissue, usually a tumor, or other small lesion using cutting instruments or electrosurgery.

11. _____ this refers to an undesirable pucker in skin as a result of poor suture placement.

12. _____ In surgical terms, this means to "bring together" tissues by suturing or other means.

a. Amputate

b. Anastomose

c. Approximate

d. Blunt dissection

e. Debridement

f. Dog ear

g. Debulk

h. Dissect

i. Elevate

j. Excise

k. Exteriorize

l. Ligate

MATCHING

Match each person with the correct job.

1. _____ Unsterile team member

2. _____ Responsible for labeling the surgical specimen

3. _____ Adjusts the surgical lights as needed during the procedure

4. _____ Escorts the patient to the operating room from preop holding

5. _____ Opens the sterile supplies onto the sterile field as the room is being opened

6. _____ Performs the surgical scrub, and gowns and gloves themselves

7. _____ Involved in the TIMEOUT

8. _____ Responsible for maintaining a clean and orderly instrument table and sterile field

9. _____ Handles and passes instruments

10. _____ Initiates the use of a neutral zone

11. _____ Signs the surgical count sheet

12. _____ Does the surgical count

13. _____ Documents the surgical proceedings

14. _____ Looks for a missing sponge

15. _____ Directly responsible for receiving and handling specimens on the surgical field

16. _____ Requests additional equipment as needed

17. _____ Directs the surgical team during an emergency

a. Scrubbed Surgical Technologist

b. Circulator

c. Surgeon

d. All team members

e. Scrubbed Surgical Technologist and circulator

MULTIPLE CHOICE

Choose the most correct answer to complete the question or statement.

1. Which of the following specimens might be sent to the pathologist on a Telfa sponge?
   a. Adenoid tissue
   b. Prostate from a transurethral resection of the prostate (TURP)
   c. Uterus and fallopian tubes
   d. Breast tissue for frozen section

2. Which of the following specimens must be sent to the pathologist dry?
   a. Colon polyps
   b. Bronchial washings
   c. Kidney stones
   d. Tonsils

3. Excessive or rough handling of bowel tissue can cause a sympathetic nervous response called _____.
   a. Paralytic ileus
   b. Small bowel obstruction
   c. Ulcerative colitis
   d. Diverticulitis

4. _____ instruments are passed firmly.
   a. Ophthalmic surgery
   b. Orthopedic surgery
   c. Plastic surgery
   d. General surgery

5. Which sponge is used to make a sponge stick?
   a. Laparotomy
   b. 4 × 4
   c. Kittner
   d. Tonsil

Chapter **21 Case Planning and Intraoperative Routine**

6. Which type of sponge is packaged in groups of 10?
   a. Kittner
   b. Cherry
   c. 4 × 4
   d. Laparotomy

7. Which type of sponge would be appropriate for "packing" the abdominal cavity?
   a. Kittner
   b. 4 × 4
   c. Laparotomy
   d. Neuro patties

8. Case planning combines knowledge of:
   a. Surgical procedure and surgical techniques
   b. Anatomy and pathology
   c. The patient's diagnosis
   d. The patient's prognosis

9. When opening packages sealed with tape, why should you break the tape rather than tear it?
   a. To prevent the outer wrapper from ripping, causing contamination
   b. So that you have to look at the tape to see whether it is sterile
   c. To prevent strike-through
   d. To prevent the inner wrapper from ripping

10. Which of the following is *not* a recommendation for opening a case?
    a. Open the scrubbed surgical technologist's gown and gloves on a small table or Mayo stand.
    b. Never unwrap a heavy item by holding it in midair.
    c. Do not open small sterile items into the genesis instrument tray.
    d. Open extra sutures, special equipment, and implants so that the surgeon does not have to wait for them during the procedure.

11. After the case has been opened, the surgical technologist's next immediate task is to:
    a. Load the knife blade
    b. Dress the Mayo stand
    c. Perform a surgical hand scrub
    d. Organize the instruments

12. Creating a continuous sterile field:
    a. Makes the instruments easy for the surgeon to reach
    b. Contaminates the back table
    c. Saves steps and motion
    d. Is against the Association of Perioperative Registered Nurses (AORN) standards

13. After finishing the surgical scrub, which task is done next?
    a. Arrange towels, gowns, and gloves in order of use
    b. Gown and glove self
    c. Organize the knife and the instruments
    d. Put all sponges in one location so you are ready to count

14. The selection of suture material is almost always prescriptive, or
    a. Written on the surgeon's case plan ahead of time
    b. Delayed until the surgeon can prescribe the type she wants
    c. Determined only after the surgeon has taken a look at the surgical wound
    d. Delayed until the surgeon has discussed surgical wound closure with the patient.

15. If the count is incorrect:
    a. A radiograph should be taken immediately.
    b. The surgeon should not be bothered.
    c. The surgeon is notified and the count repeated.
    d. The circulator should call the house supervisor for an incident report.

16. A retained item can cause patient injury from all of the following, *except:*
    a. X-ray exposure sickness
    b. Infection
    c. Organ perforation
    d. Obstruction

17. Immediately after gowning and gloving, the technologist must complete:
    a. Scattering the case
    b. The sterile setup or setting up a case
    c. Preparation of the operating room
    d. The surgical count

18. After you scrub and as you first approach the pile of sterile equipment, do not move anything until:
    a. You have a plan.
    b. You count the instruments.
    c. You load the blade on the knife handle.
    d. You move the drapes and put them in order.

CASE STUDIES

1. *Read the following case study and answer the questions based on your knowledge of case preparation.*

   It is 6:30 AM, and you are assigned to operating room 6 with your preceptor, who has called and said that she will be late because she has a flat tire. She has asked that you go ahead and get the room ready for the day, "pick the case," and then "scatter the room" (which is to place the sterile, but unopened, packs onto the furniture where they will be opened soon). She does not want you to "open the case" until she gets there to assist you.

   a. How do you get the room "ready" for the day?

   b. What is involved in "picking the case"?

   c. What are you going to do to "scatter the room"?

   d. Why does your preceptor *not* want you to open the case until she is present?

2. *Read the following case study and answer the questions based on your knowledge of case preparation.*

Think about putting yourself in the surgical technologist's role. Your surgeon has just come in, and you are about to hand him the towel. What is the sequence of events between that sterile towel and the incision?

1. Towels are distributed, and the team members are gowned and gloved.

2.

3.

4.

5.

6.

7. The incision is made.

SKILLS PERFORMANCE CHECKLIST: SUTURE/NEEDLE/STAPLE HANDLING—LOAD, PASS, AND UNLOAD A NEEDLE HOLDER USING THE DIRECT PASSING TECHNIQUE

Student's Name: _____ Date: _____

Task: Student demonstrates the ability to properly load suture material and safely pass suture to surgeon.

Equipment and Supplies:

- Proper suture
- Appropriate needle holder
- Appropriate additional instruments (forceps, scissors, or both)

Evaluation Directions: Check or circle the appropriate number to indicate the student's performance level, using the following rating scale.

3-PROFICIENT. Can complete the task quickly and accurately without direction.

2-PARTIALLY PROFICIENT. Can do most of the task. Needs assistance. Needs constant supervision.

1-LIMITED. Can do a limited amount of the task. Must be told what to do. Needs extremely close supervision.

0-UNSATISFACTORY. Can do a limited amount of the task. Must be told what to do. Needs extremely close supervision.

Task Checklist	Rating	Self-Assessment	Instructor Assessment
1. Open suture packet	0 1 2 3		
2. Needle holder is loaded for right-handed or left-handed surgeon	0 1 2 3		
3. Pass suture to surgeon	0 1 2 3		
4. Pass additional instruments (forceps, Mayo scissors, or both)	0 1 2 3		
5. Suture needle is returned from field	0 1 2 3		
6. Needle holder is reloaded or returned to proper place	0 1 2 3		
Total Score			

SCORE

18-15 = A

14-11 = B

10-8 = C

Below 8 = not passing

Comments:

_____

_____

_____

_____

Student's Name: _____ Date: _____

Task: Students will apply knowledge they have learned in the classroom to the lab setting.

Equipment and Supplies:

- Scrub brushes
- Gowns
- Gloves
- Drapes
- Back table cover
- Instruments
- Accessory supplies

Evaluation Directions: Check or circle the appropriate number to indicate the student's performance level, using the following rating scale:

3-PROFICIENT. Can complete the task quickly and accurately without direction.

2-PARTIALLY PROFICIENT. Can do most of the task. Needs assistance. Needs constant supervision.

1-LIMITED. Can do a limited amount of the task. Must be told what to do. Needs extremely close supervision.

0-UNSATISFACTORY. Can do a limited amount of the task. Must be told what to do. Needs extremely close supervision.

Task Checklist	Rating	Self-Assessment	Instructor Assessment
1. Break down sterile field.	0 1 2 3		
2. Check drapes and floor for instruments.	0 1 2 3		
3. Dispose of single use items.	0 1 2 3		
4. Dispose of sharps and glass in appropriate containers.	0 1 2 3		
5. Remove trash and lines from operating room.	0 1 2 3		
6. Perform terminal sterilization of instruments, basin, trays, etc.	0 1 2 3		
7. Clean contaminated furniture and floor of operating room.	0 1 2 3		

Task Checklist	Rating	Self-Assessment	Instructor Assessment
8. Stock cabinets in operating room.	0 1 2 3		
9. Maintain fast turnover time and prepare for the next case	0 1 2 3		
Total Score			

SCORE

27-25 = A

24-22 = B

21-19 = C

Below 19 = not passing

Comments:

_____

_____

_____

_____

Student's Name: _____ Date: _____

Task: Students will apply classroom theory to lab theory.

Equipment and Supplies:

- Hats
- Mask
- Shoe covers
- Sterile packs
- Instruments

Evaluation Directions: Check or circle the appropriate number to indicate the student's performance level, using the following rating scale:

3-PROFICIENT. Can complete the task quickly and accurately without direction.

2-PARTIALLY PROFICIENT. Can do most of the task. Needs assistance. Needs constant supervision.

1-LIMITED. Can do a limited amount of the task. Must be told what to do. Needs extremely close supervision.

0-UNSATISFACTORY. Can do a limited amount of the task. Must be told what to do. Needs extremely close supervision.

Task Checklist	Rating	Self-Assessment	Instructor Assessment
1. Don mask, shoe covers, hat, and surgical scrubs	0 1 2 3		
2. Damp-dust lights and other furniture	0 1 2 3		
3. Organize room by arranging furniture and equipment	0 1 2 3		
4. Check function of basic and specialty equipment	0 1 2 3		
5. Remove and report defective or inoperable furniture and equipment	0 1 2 3		
6. Check surgeon's preference card	0 1 2 3		
7. Gather instruments, supplies, positioning devices, and equipment for case	0 1 2 3		
8. Place packs on appropriate furniture	0 1 2 3		

Task Checklist	Rating	Self-Assessment	Instructor Assessment
9. Opening sterile supplies	0 1 2 3		
a. Identify basic supplies	0 1 2 3		
b. Check sterility indicators	0 1 2 3		
c. Place packs and instruments on proper operating room furniture (backtable-backtable cover, basin-ring stand, instrument-ring stand, or small table)	0 1 2 3		
d. Open packs using aseptic technique (check sterility indicators)	0 1 2 3		
e. Open packs as close as possible to the time of surgery	0 1 2 3		
f. Dispense supplies to sterile field (using proper technique-flip)	0 1 2 3		
10. Before surgical scrub			
a. Remove jewelry	0 1 2 3		
b. Secure mask and protective eyewear	0 1 2 3		
c. Open gown and gloves (on proper operating room furniture [i.e., prep stand])	0 1 2 3		
11. Surgical hand scrub (using both the count method and timed method)			
a. Preliminary wash and rinse	0 1 2 3		
b. Open brush package	0 1 2 3		
c. Antiseptic agents	0 1 2 3		
d. Timed method (well-executed scrub is 3 to 5 minutes)	0 1 2 3		
e. Brush-stroke method	0 1 2 3		
f. Elevate hands	0 1 2 3		
g. Scrub from fingertips to 2 inches above elbows	0 1 2 3		
h. Final rinse	0 1 2 3		
12. Drying your hands and arms using aseptic technique	0 1 2 3		
13. Gowning (self)	0 1 2 3		
14. Gloving (open method and closed gloved method)	0 1 2 3		

Task Checklist	Rating	Self-Assessment	Instructor Assessment
15. Gowning and gloving team members	0 1 2 3		
16. Remove gown and gloves	0 1 2 3		
Total Score			

SCORE

90-81 = A

80-72 = B

71-63 = C

Below 63 = not passing

Comments:

_____

_____

_____

_____

Student's Name: _____ Date: _____

Task: Students will apply classroom knowledge to lab skills.

Equipment and Supplies:

- Operating room attire
- Back table covers
- Instruments
- Drapes
- Basin
- Sterile supplies
- Scrub brush
- Gown
- Gloves
- Any other items.

Evaluation Directions: Check or circle the appropriate number to indicate the student's performance level, using the following rating scale:

3-PROFICIENT. Can complete the task quickly and accurately without direction.

2-PARTIALLY PROFICIENT. Can do most of the task. Needs assistance. Needs constant supervision.

1-LIMITED. Can do a limited amount of the task. Must be told what to do. Needs extremely close supervision.

0-UNSATISFACTORY. Can do a limited amount of the task. Must be told what to do. Needs extremely close supervision.

Task Checklist	Rating	Self-Assessment	Instructor Assessment
1. Preparation of case-pull supplies/ equipment	0 1 2 3		
2. Preparation of case-opening/clean up	0 1 2 3		
3. Applies principles of aseptic technique	0 1 2 3		
4. Observes Universal Precautions	0 1 2 3		
5. Scrubbing, gowning, and gloving	0 1 2 3		
6. Team gowning, and gloving	0 1 2 3		
7. Draping (with help)	0 1 2 3		
8. Anticipation passing of instruments	0 1 2 3		
9. Prepares/assist in applying dressing	0 1 2 3		

Task Checklist	Rating	Self-Assessment	Instructor Assessment
10. Sterile setup			
a. Mayo	0 1 2 3		
b. Back table	0 1 2 3		
11. Counts			
a. Sponges	0 1 2 3		
b. Needles	0 1 2 3		
c. Instruments	0 1 2 3		
12. Behavior			
a. Punctuality	0 1 2 3		
b. Functions as a team member (pre-intra-post-op)	0 1 2 3		
c. Follows directions	0 1 2 3		
d. Attitude	0 1 2 3		
13. Work ethic			
a. Attendance	0 1 2 3		
b. Efficient use of time	0 1 2 3		
c. Personal appearance in health care setting	0 1 2 3		
Total Score			

SCORE

63-57 = A

56-51 = B

50-44 = C

Below 44 = not passing

Comments:

_____

_____

_____

_____

Student's Name: _____ Date: _____

Task: Students will apply knowledge they have learned in the classroom to the lab setting.

Equipment and Supplies:

- Scrub brushes
- Gowns
- Gloves
- Drapes
- Back table cover
- Instruments
- Accessory supplies

Evaluation Directions: Check or circle the appropriate number to indicate the student's performance level, using the following rating scale:

3-PROFICIENT. Can complete the task quickly and accurately without direction.

2-PARTIALLY PROFICIENT. Can do most of the task. Needs assistance. Needs constant supervision.

1-LIMITED. Can do a limited amount of the task. Must be told what to do. Needs extremely close supervision.

0-UNSATISFACTORY. Can do a limited amount of the task. Must be told what to do. Needs extremely close supervision.

Task Checklist	Rating	Self-Assessment	Instructor Assessment
1. Pass scalpels			
a. Left handed surgeon	0 1 2 3		
b. Right handed surgeon	0 1 2 3		
c. Neutral zone	0 1 2 3		
2. Pass instruments (both left and right handed surgeon)	0 1 2 3		
3. Prepare and pass sutures (both left and right handed surgeon)	0 1 2 3		
4. Pass sponges as needed	0 1 2 3		
5. Receive medications on sterile field (use medication check off list)	0 1 2 3		
6. Pass irrigating solutions to surgeon	0 1 2 3		

Task Checklist	Rating	Self-Assessment	Instructor Assessment
7. Discard contaminated items	0 1 2 3		
8. Receive sterile items from the circulator	0 1 2 3		
9. Receive specimens from the surgeon	0 1 2 3		
10. Dispense specimens to circulator	0 1 2 3		
11. Maintain sterile field	0 1 2 3		
12. Maintain counts throughout the procedure	0 1 2 3		
13. Care for instruments throughout the procedure	0 1 2 3		
14. Prepare and pass medications to surgeon	0 1 2 3		
15. Count sponges and instruments	0 1 2 3		
Total Score			

SCORE

51-46 = A

45-41 = B

40-36 = C

Below 36 = not passing

Comments:

_____

_____

_____

_____

SKILLS PERFORMANCE CHECKLIST: SUTURE/NEEDLE/STAPLE HANDLING—LOAD, PASS, AND UNLOAD A NEEDLE HOLDER USING THE NEUTRAL ZONE TECHNIQUE

Student's Name: _____ Date: _____

Task: Student demonstrates knowledge of utilizing neutral zone when passing loaded needle drivers.

Equipment and Supplies:

- Proper suture
- Appropriate needle driver
- Appropriate additional instruments (forceps, scissors)
- Magnetic needle box

Evaluation Directions: Check or circle the appropriate number to indicate the student's performance level, using the following rating scale:

3-PROFICIENT. Can complete the task quickly and accurately without direction.

2-PARTIALLY PROFICIENT. Can do most of the task. Needs assistance. Needs constant supervision.

1-LIMITED. Can do a limited amount of the task. Must be told what to do. Needs extremely close supervision.

0-UNSATISFACTORY. Can do a limited amount of the task. Must be told what to do. Needs extremely close supervision.

Task Checklist	Rating	Self-Assessment	Instructor Assessment
1. Open suture packet	0 1 2 3		
2. Needle driver is loading using "no-touch" technique.	0 1 2 3		
3. Loaded needle driver is placed in the neutral zone for right-handed or left-handed surgeon.	0 1 2 3		
4. Appropriate instrument (forceps or scissors) is passed to surgeon.	0 1 2 3		
5. Needle driver is retrieved from the neutral zone.	0 1 2 3		
6. Suture needle is placed in magnetic needle box.	0 1 2 3		
Total Score			

SCORE

18-15 = A

14-11 = B

10-8 = C

Below 8 = not passing

Comments:

_____

_____

_____

_____

22 Management of the Surgical Wound

Student's Name _____

KEY TERMS

Write the definition for each term.

1. Absorbable suture: _____

2. Adhesion: _____

3. Anastomosis: _____

4. Approximate: _____

5. Autotransfusion: _____

6. Capillary action: _____

7. Contracture: _____

8. Debridement: _____

9. Dehiscence: _____

10. Evisceration: _____

11. Fistula: _____

12. Hematoma: _____

13. Hemostatic agent: _____

14. Inert: _____

15. Interrupted sutures: _____

16. Ligate: _____

17. Nonabsorbable suture: _____

18. Primary intention: _____

19. Running suture: _____

20. Serosanguineous fluid: _____

21. Swage: _____

22. Tapered needle: _____

23. Tensile strength: _____

24. Throw: _____

25. Tie on a passer: _____

SHORT ANSWERS

Provide a short answer for each question or statement.

1. List the primary features in wound healing.

   _____

   _____

2. List Halstead's principles of surgery and define.

   a. _____

   b. _____

   c. _____

   d. _____

   e. _____

   f. _____

3. What are four primary techniques of hemostasis used in surgery?

   a. _____

   b. _____

   c. _____

   d. _____

4. What are the guidelines for placement of a surgical tourniquet?

   _____

   _____

5. What physical injury can be done to the surgical patient if a surgical tourniquet is not used properly?

_____

_____

6. All substances, including suture products, that bear the USP label must meet minimum standards. What are the standards for sutures?

_____

_____

7. List the five characteristics of sutures that influence a surgeon's decision in choosing a suture.

a. _____

b. _____

c. _____

d. _____

e. _____

8. List all the suture materials that have *no* inflammatory properties.

_____

_____

9. Describe the types of suture needles.

_____

_____

10. The following is a list of names of alternate and not well known, or infrequently used, grafting materials. Explain what each is and the purpose for which it is used.

a. Amniotic membrane

_____

b. Engineered skin substitutes

_____

c. Biobrane

_____

d. TransCyte

_____

e. Integra Bilayer Matrix Wound Dressing

_____

f. Integra Dermal Regeneration Template

_____

g. Cultured epithelial autograft

_____

h. Foreskin grafts

_____

i. What are the purposes of wound dressings?

_____

LABELING

Label the following pictures with the type of suture technique shown.

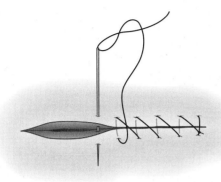

1. _____

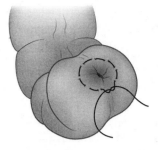

3. _____

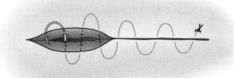

2. _____

MATCHING

Match each term with the correct definition as it applies to implants and grafts.

1. _____ Tissue used to cover large defects in the skin

2. _____ Any type of tissue replacement or device placed in the body

3. _____ Tissue graft derived from human tissue

4. _____ Graft taken from pig tissue

5. _____ Tissue obtained from the patient's body and implanted in another site

6. _____ Graft taken from a species different from that of the patient

7. _____ Migration of epithelial cells into the wound during healing

8. _____ Graft taken from beef origin

a. Allograft

b. Autograft

c. Bovine graft

d. Epithelialization

e. Implant

f. Porcine graft

g. Xenograft

h. Wound cover

MATCHING

Match each term with the correct definition as it applies to hemostatic drugs and agents. You may use the same answer more than once.

1. _____ When applied to oozing tissue, this product combines with fibrinogen to promote coagulation.

2. _____ This product is used on bleeding bone.

3. _____ This product may be soaked in normal saline or topical thrombin or used in dry form.

4. _____ The brand name of this product is Surgicel.

5. _____ This powder is applied directly to an oozing surface or mixed with injectable isotonic saline for use as a spray or for soaking hemostatic sponges.

6. _____ This product is never injected into blood vessels.

7. _____ When applied to tissue, this product absorbs blood quickly and forms an artificial clot.

8. _____ This product is available in squares that are cut to size as needed.

9. _____ The unused pieces of this product must be kept away from the surgical wound.

10. _____ The brand name of this product is Avitene.

11. _____ This product is available in mesh.

12. _____ This product must be warmed slightly before use.

a. Thrombin

b. Absorbable gelatin

c. Oxidized cellulose

d. Collagen absorbable hemostat

e. Bone wax

MULTIPLE CHOICE

Choose the most correct answer to complete the question or statement.

1. Conserving the body's total blood volume necessary for life is called:
   a. Coagulation
   b. Ligation
   c. Homeostasis
   d. Hemostasis

2. Uncontrolled oozing or insecure hemostasis can lead to a:
   a. Hematoma
   b. Contusion
   c. Seroma
   d. Compartment syndrome

3. Which of the following statements is true regarding the formation of a clot?
   a. The blood vessel retracts and constricts.
   b. Even in severe trauma, the body's natural mechanisms control bleeding.
   c. A meshwork of fibrin strands forms around the blood cells.
   d. Once initiated, the clotting cascade takes one route to form a clot.

4. Collection of the patient's blood from the surgical site intraoperatively and intravenous return of the blood is called:
   a. Coagulation
   b. Autotransfusion
   c. Hemostasis
   d. Cell Saver

5. Suture materials are used for all of the following, *except:*
   a. Approximation
   b. Ligation of tubular structures
   c. Hemostasis
   d. Coagulation

6. Which of the following is the *largest* suture type?
   a. # 1 Ethibond
   b. # 0 silk
   c. 3-0 Vicryl
   d. 11-0 chromic

7. The physical characteristics of a suture include which of the following?
   a. Size
   b. Elasticity
   c. Memory
   d. Effect of the suture on the tissue

8. Which of the following suture terms indicates multiple intertwined strands?
   a. Monofilament
   b. Multifilament
   c. Braided
   d. Twisted

9. The _____ of suture refers to the amount of force needed to break the suture.
   a. Knot strength
   b. Tensile strength
   c. Tissue drag
   d. Biological environment

10. Which type of suture is absorbed rapidly in the presence of infection and is not used in contaminated wounds?
    a. Silk
    b. Vicryl
    c. Ethibond
    d. Chromic

11. _____ sutures are no longer marketed in the United States because they have been replaced by more inert materials.
    a. Silk
    b. Cotton
    c. Chromic
    d. Biosyn

12. A wound that is not sutured and must heal from the base is healing by: _____
    a. Delayed union
    b. First intention
    c. Secondary intention
    d. Third intention

13. Which of the following is the first phase of wound healing?
    a. Healing phase
    b. Remodeling phase
    c. Proliferative phase
    d. Inflammatory phase

14. Which of the following is *not* considered a risk factor in wound healing?
    a. Nutritional status
    b. Chronic disease
    c. Obesity
    d. Site of the incision

15. Tissue breakdown at the wound margins is called: _____
    a. Dehiscence
    b. Evisceration
    c. Enucleation
    d. Surgical wound infection

CASE STUDIES

1. *Read the following case study and answer the question based on your knowledge of surgical tourniquets.*

   Your surgical patient is going to arrive at the operating room soon for a total knee replacement. You know that the surgeon will require a surgical tourniquet for the procedure. What safeguards are in place to keep your patient safe during the time the tourniquet is being placed and used?

2. *Making a suture square: Using the squares below, categorize the sutures from the text. After you have finished that, use a colored pencil to make the suture name in the same color as the suture package.*

	Synthetic Sutures	Natural Sutures
Absorbable sutures		
Nonabsorbable sutures		

SKILLS PERFORMANCE CHECKLIST: INSTRUMENT HANDLING—LOAD, PASS, AND UNLOAD A SCALPEL HANDLE

Student's Name: _____ Date: _____

Task: Student demonstrates knowledge of using neutral zone when passing scalpels.

Equipment and Supplies:

- Scalpel blade
- Knife handle
- Needle driver
- Sharps container

Evaluation Directions: Check or circle the appropriate number to indicate the student's performance level, using the following rating scale:

3-PROFICIENT. Can complete the task quickly and accurately without direction.

2-PARTIALLY PROFICIENT. Can do most of the task. Needs assistance. Needs constant supervision.

1-LIMITED. Can do a limited amount of the task. Must be told what to do. Needs extremely close supervision.

0-UNSATISFACTORY. Can do a limited amount of the task. Must be told what to do. Needs extremely close supervision.

Task Checklist	Rating	Self-Assessment	Instructor Assessment
1. Scalpel blade is secured using needle driver.	0 1 2 3		
2. Blade is applied to handle using needle driver.	0 1 2 3		
3. Scalpel is placed in a designated neutral zone.	0 1 2 3		
4. Scalpel is retrieved from neutral zone.	0 1 2 3		
5. Blade is removed from handle using a needle driver.	0 1 2 3		
6. Dispose of blade properly.	0 1 2 3		
Total Score			

SCORE

18-15 = A

14-11 = B

10-8 = C

Below 8 = not passing

Comments:

_____

_____

_____

_____

SKILLS PERFORMANCE CHECKLIST: SUTURE/NEEDLE/STAPLE HANDLING—PASS TIES (INCLUDES REEL, FREE TIES, AND TIES ON A PASS)

Student's Name: _____ Date: _____

Task: Student demonstrates knowledge of passing sutures for ties.

Equipment and Supplies:

- Suture material of various types
- Scissors
- Passer instrument (Mixter, hemostat)

Evaluation Directions: Check or circle the appropriate number to indicate the student's performance level, using the following rating scale:

3-PROFICIENT. Can complete the task quickly and accurately without direction.

2-PARTIALLY PROFICIENT. Can do most of the task. Needs assistance. Needs constant supervision.

1-LIMITED. Can do a limited amount of the task. Must be told what to do. Needs extremely close supervision.

0-UNSATISFACTORY. Can do a limited amount of the task. Must be told what to do. Needs extremely close supervision.

Task Checklist	Rating	Self-Assessment	Instructor Assessment
1. Select necessary suture	0 1 2 3		
2. Prepare and pass a free tie	0 1 2 3		
3. Prepare and pass tie on a passer	0 1 2 3		
4. Pass scissors	0 1 2 3		
Total Score			

12-10 = A

9-7 = B

6-4 = C

Below 4 = not passing

Comments: _____

_____

_____

_____

_____

Chapter **22 Management of the Surgical Wound**

Label the axillary anatomy of the breast.

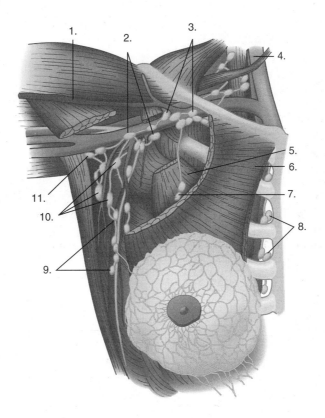

1. _____
2. _____
3. _____
4. _____
5. _____
6. _____

7. _____
8. _____
9. _____
10. _____
11. _____

Label the biliary and hepatic anatomy.

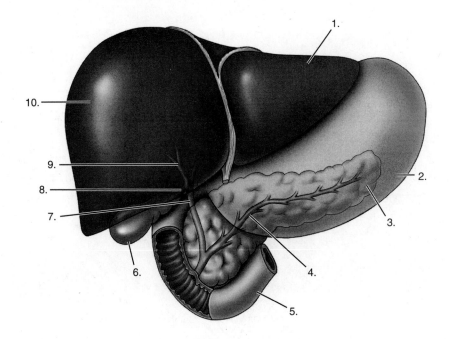

1. _____
2. _____
3. _____
4. _____
5. _____

6. _____
7. _____
8. _____
9. _____
10. _____

Draw in the following types of abdominal incisions.

1. Subcostal

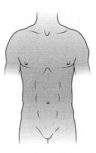

2. Paramedian

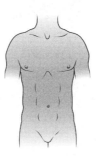

3. McBurney

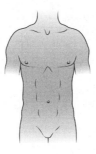

4. Pfannenstiel

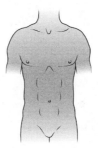

5. Upper midline

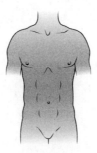

6. Upper abdominal transverse

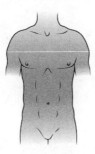

7. Oblique

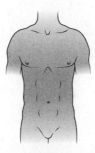

8. Lower midline

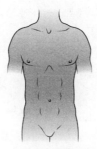

CASE STUDIES

1. *You are scrubbed in on an emergency endoscopic appendectomy. What are the exact eight steps (in order) for performing an appendectomy?*

   a. _____

   b. _____

   c. _____

   d. _____

   e. _____

   f. _____

   g. _____

   h. _____

Student's Name _____

KEY TERMS

Write the definition for each term.

1. Active electrode monitoring (AEM): _____

2. Arthroscopy: _____

3. Auxiliary water channel: _____

4. Biopsy channel: _____

5. Camera control unit (CCU): _____

6. Cannula: _____

7. Capacitative coupling: _____

8. Control head: _____

9. Diagnostic endoscopy: _____

10. Digital output recorder: _____

11. Direct coupling: _____

12. Docking: _____

13. Elevator channel: _____

14. Endocoupler: _____

15. Extracorporeal: _____

16. Gain: _____

17. Haptic feedback: _____

18. High definition (HD): _____

19. Imaging system: _____

20. Insertion tube: _____

21. Instrument channel: _____

22. Insufflation: _____

23. Intracorporeal: _____

24. Intravasation: _____

25. Knot pusher: _____

26. Ligation loop: _____

27. Light cable: _____

28. Light source: _____

29. Master controllers: _____

30. Optical angle: _____

31. Pixel: _____

32. Pneumoperitoneum: _____

33. Resectoscope: _____

34. Robot: _____

35. Standard definition (SD): _____

36. Stereoscopic viewer: _____

37. Telesurgery: _____

38. Veress needle: _____

39. Video cable: _____

40. Video printer: _____

41. White balance: _____

SHORT ANSWER

Provide a short answer for each question or statement.

1. Describe the difference between rigid endoscopy and flexible endoscopy.

   _____

   _____

2. What are the advantages to the patient with MIS?

   _____

   _____

3. What are the limitations associated with MIS?

_____

_____

4. What are the special considerations when prepping and draping for MIS procedures?

_____

_____

5. What are the components of the surgical imaging system?

_____

_____

6. The guidelines for taking care of the fiberoptic cables include:

   a. _____

   b. _____

   c. _____

   d. _____

   e. _____

   f. _____

   g. _____

7. What is the procedure for white balancing?

_____

_____

8. Describe the process of insufflation.

_____

_____

9. What is the procedure for insertion of a Veress needle?

_____

_____

10. During which procedures would continuous irrigation be used?

_____

_____

11. What are the guidelines for precleaning optical parts and lenses?

_____

_____

MATCHING

Match each term with the correct definition. You may use the same answer more than once.

1. _____ In minimally invasive surgery, the inflation of the abdominal or thoracic cavity with carbon dioxide gas.

2. _____ Refers to the abdomen when it is distended with carbon dioxide gas.

3. _____ In laparoscopic surgery, a type of cannula that is secured to the abdominal wall with sutures.

4. _____ Meaning "outside the body."

5. _____ A device that controls and emits light for delivery in endoscopic procedures.

6. _____ A sharp, rod-shaped instrument used to puncture the body wall.

7. _____ A surgical technique in which tissue is fragmented to permit removal through an endoscopic cannula.

8. _____ Long, narrow instruments used during endoscopic surgery.

9. _____ A hollow tube

10. _____ A spring-loaded needle used to deliver carbon dioxide gas during insufflation.

11. _____ A commercially prepared suture loop used to secure structures during minimally invasive surgery.

12. _____ The fiberoptic light cable that transmits light from the source to the endoscopic instrument.

13. _____ Refers to the rigid lensed instrument used in minimally invasive surgery.

14. _____ Instrument passed through a natural orifice for assessment or surgery of a hollow organ, duct, or vessel.

a. Light source

b. Light cable

c. Endoscope

d. Cannula

e. Hasson cannula

f. Telescopic instruments

g. Extracorporeal

h. Veress needle

i. Insufflation

j. Pneumoperitoneum

k. Trocar

l. Ligation loop

m. Morcellation

CASE STUDIES

1. *You are scrubbed in on a laparoscopic procedure that is about to finish. Your responsibility as a surgical technologist is to properly handle and care for the laparoscope. What does that include?*

   a. _____

   b. _____

   c. _____

   d. _____

   e. _____

2. *Your surgical patient is undergoing a hysteroscopy. As an educated scrub tech, you know that you must use only nonconductive, salt-free fluids for the continuous irrigation that will be required to perform the procedure.*

   a. What solutions might your surgeon choose to meet these qualifications?

   b. One of the risks involved in these procedures is intravasation. What is intravasation?

Chapter **24** **Minimally Invasive Endoscopic and Robotic-Assisted Surgery**

c. What injury is involved in intravasation?

d. Who is responsible for keeping track of the fluid inflow and output in these procedures?

f. Current medications and allergies

g. Family history

h. Social history

2. *Gynecology procedures are performed with the patient in the supine or lithotomy position. What are the critical safety considerations for the lithotomy position?*

  a. _____

  b. _____

  c. _____

  d. _____

  e. _____

  f. _____

  g. _____

3. *You are scrubbed on a laparoscopic tubal ligation, please answer the following questions:*

    a. Define laparoscopic tubal ligation.

    b. What position will the patient be in?

    c. What instrument trays will you use?

    d. What type of prep will be used?

    e. How will you drape?

f. What type of setup will you use?

g. What anatomy do you need to be aware of?

CASE STUDIES

1. *You are about to scrub for a cystoscopy when the operating room supervisor delivers a surgical technology student to you and asks you to serve as her preceptor for the case. Your student has never seen a cystoscopy before, and you decide to describe the procedure to her before you start. What steps would you describe to her to explain the procedure?*

   a.

   b.

   c.

   d.

   e.

f.

g.

h.

2. *During cystoscopic procedures, the bladder is distended with fluid to enhance visualization of the internal structures. Describe the following solutions, which are commonly used in cystoscopic procedures, and explain when they might be used.*

a. Sorbitol

b. Glycine

b. Now color code the sets of muscles.

c. During an R&R, which muscle is resected?

d. Which muscle is regressed?

2. *You are about to scrub for a left cataract extraction with an intraocular lens (IOL). What is the protocol for implantation of an IOL?*

The protocol includes:

a.

b.

c.

d.

Provide a short answer for each question or statement.

1. List the structures of the larynx.

_____

_____

2. What is the normal patient position for ear, nose, and throat (ENT) procedures?

_____

_____

3. List the diagnostic procedures of the ear and define.

_____

_____

4. List the equipment, supplies, and medication needed for an ear procedure.

_____

_____

5. How does the ear prep and draping differ from a thyroidectomy?

_____

_____

MATCHING I

Match each term with the correct definition. (Choices may be used more than once or not at all.)

1. _____ A benign tumor of the middle ear caused by shedding of keratin in chronic otitis media

2. _____ Defect that can be caused by a blast injury or penetrating foreign body in the ear

3. _____ Enlargement of the tonsils that may prevent swallowing

4. _____ A benign epithelial tumor characterized by a branching or lobular shape

5. _____ Fluid in the middle ear

6. _____ Bleeding arising from the nasal cavity

7. _____ Vibration of the vocal cords during speaking or vocalization

8. _____ The most common cause of a break in the ossicle chain, which erodes the ossicles

9. _____ Paralysis of a structure, such as vocal cord paresis

10. _____ Excessive proliferation of mucosal epithelium

11. _____ Hearing impairment arising from the cochlea, auditory nerve, or central nervous system

12. _____ Abnormal thickening of the bone in the middle and inner ear

a. Cholesteatoma

b. Papilloma

c. Polyp

d. Perforation

e. Epistaxis

f. Effusion

g. Hypertrophy

h. Paresis

i. Sensorineural hearing loss

j. Nystagmus

k. Phonation

l. Otosclerosis

MATCHING II

Match each term with the correct definition.

1. _____ A surgical opening is made in the tympanic membrane to release fluid

2. _____ Close a small, nonhealing hole in the tympanic membrane

3. _____ Surgical removal of a cholesteatoma and mastoid bone, with or without reconstruction

4. _____ Removal of diseased bone, the mastoid air cells, and the soft tissue lining the air cell of the mastoid

5. _____ The reconstruction of the ossicles to restore conduction to the oval window.

6. _____ Is used to transmit external sound directly to the VIII cranial nerve

a. Mastoidectomy/tympanomastoidectomy

b. Cochlear implant

c. Myringotomy

d. Tympanoplasty

e. Stapedectomy/ossicular reconstruction

f. Myringoplasty

SHORT ANSWER

Provide a short answer for each question or statement.

1. List the anatomy of the larynx.

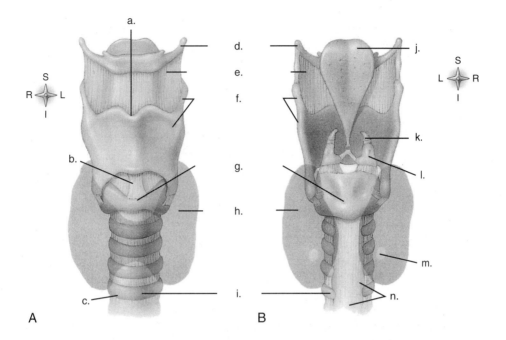

A   B

a. _____

b. _____

c. _____

d. _____

e. _____

f. _____

g. _____

h. _____

i. _____

j. _____

k. _____

l. _____

m. _____

n. _____

2. List the diagnostic tests associated with nasal cavity, oropharynx, and larynx surgery.

_____

_____

3. List the equipment, supplies, and medication needed for ear, nose, and throat (ENT) surgery.

_____

_____

4. Give an example of the following nasal instruments and define:

a. Retractors

_____

_____

b. Knives

_____

_____

c. Elevator or dissector

_____

_____

d. Forceps

_____

_____

e. Rongeur

_____

_____

f. Gouge, chisel, and osteotome

_____

_____

g. Rasp and saw

_____

_____

5. List the tonsil and adenoid instruments.

_____

_____

MATCHING

Match each term with the correct definition.

1. _____ Is performed to treat disease of the paranasal sinus, nasal cavity, and skull base and to improve nasal airflow

2. _____ Maxillary sinus is exposed by making an incision in the gingival-buccal sulcus

3. _____ Removal of the bony turbinate to increase airflow through the nose

4. _____ Surgical manipulation of the septum to return it to the correct anatomical position or to gain access to the sphenoid sinus for removal of a pituitary tumor

5. _____ Is performed to reshape the external nose for aesthetic or functional purposes

6. _____ Is performed to eradicate infection, improve the airway, or remove a cancer

7. _____ Surgical removal of the adenoids

8. _____ Performed to reduce and tighten oropharyngeal tissue

9. _____ Endoscopic assessment of the larynx

10. _____ Is performed to provide patient airway

a. Septoplasty

b. Endoscopic sinus surgery (ESS)

c. Tracheostomy/tracheostomy

d. Tonsillectomy

e. Caldwell-Luc

f. Laryngoscopy

g. Adenoidectomy

h. Turbinectomy/turbinate reduction

i. Rhinoplasty

j. UPP

LABELING

Label the structures of the neck.

1. _____

2. _____

3. _____

4. _____

5. _____

6. _____

From Potter PA, Perry AG: *Fundamentals of nursing*, ed 5, St Louis, 2001, Mosby.

SHORT ANSWER

Provide a short answer for each question or statement.

1. List the diagnostic tests associated with neck surgery.

_____

_____

2. Describe the types of dressings commonly used in neck procedures.

_____

_____

CASE STUDIES

1. *Choanal atresia is a congenital stricture of the choana that may require emergency surgery to restore respiration. Understanding the anatomy of the stricture is important to understanding the surgical procedure. Answer the following questions about choanal atresia.*

   a. What is the primary age group affected by the deformity?

b. What is the nature of the anomaly?

c. Explain the term *obligate nose breather.*

d. Describe the repair step by step.

    i.

    ii.

    iii.

    iv.

    v.

    vi.

2. *If you are about to scrub for a radical neck dissection, you will have to know the extent of the dissection or the degree of pathology. What are the three types of neck dissection? What is involved in each?*

    a.

    b.

c.

3. *You are called back in for a tonsil bleed. What are the supplies and steps necessary to perform this surgery?*

   a.

   b.

   c.

   d.

e.

f.

g.

h.

i.

j.

k.

l.

To increase your knowledge of the anatomy of the bones of the face, label the following diagram.

1. _____

2. _____

3. _____

4. _____

5. _____

6. _____

7. _____

8. _____

9. _____

10. _____

11. _____

12. _____

Modified from Thibodeau GA, Patt KT: *Anthony's textbook of anatomy and physiology*, ed 17, St Louis, 2003, Mosby.

SHORT ANSWER

Provide a short answer for each question or statement.

1. Procedures involving facial reconstruction and facial trauma involve a multidisciplinary team. Describe the team and procedure.

_____

_____

2. List the supplies, equipment, and medication needed for oral and maxillofacial surgery.

_____

_____

3. List the diagnostic tests needed for oral and maxillofacial surgery.

_____

_____

MATCHING

Match each term with the correct definition. You may use the same answer more than once or not at all.

1. _____ Realignment of the dentition of the mandible and midface

2. _____ Weight-bearing structures of the face

3. _____ Involved in "blowout" fractures

4. _____ Used to replace injured or lost dentition

5. _____ Knuckle-shaped portion of bone

6. _____ Open reduction and internal fixation of a fracture

7. _____ Procedure performed to remove teeth

a. Maxillomandibular fixation
b. ORIF
c. Buttresses
d. Condyle
e. Orbital floor
f. Frontal sinus
g. Dental implants
h. Odontectomy

CASE STUDIES

1. *Many diagrams of the midface, mandible, and other bony anatomy include the medical descriptive term, "process." What does this term indicate with regard to bone? You may have to look this up in your medical terminology text.*

2. *Your patient has a malar complex fracture. You know that for the "complex" to be mobile, five fractures must be involved. Which "cheek" bones are involved in a malar complex fracture?*

   a.

   b.

c.

d.

e.

30 Plastic and Reconstructive Surgery

Student's Name _____

Write the definition for each term.

1. Aesthetic surgery: _____

2. Allograft: _____

3. Autograft: _____

4. Biological graft: _____

5. Biosynthetic: _____

6. Composite graft: _____

7. Debridement: _____

8. Dermatome: _____

9. Eschar: _____

10. Escharotomy: _____

11. Fasciotomy: _____

12. Full-thickness skin graft (FTSG): _____

13. Hydrodressing: _____

14. Hypertrophic scar: _____

15. Implant: _____

16. Keloid: _____

17. Mohs surgery: _____

18. Photodamage: _____

19. Plication: _____

20. Porcine: _____

21. Ptosis: _____

22. Split-thickness (or partial-thickness) skin graft (STSG): _____

23. Synthetic grafts: _____

24. Undermine: _____

25. Xenograft: _____

LABELING

Label the following diagram of the epidermis.

1. _____

2. _____

3. _____

4. _____

5. _____

6. _____

7. _____

8. _____

9. _____

10. _____

11. _____

12. _____

13. _____

14. _____

15. _____

16. _____

17. _____

18. _____

From Thibodeau GA, Patton KT: *Anthony's textbook of anatomy and physiology*, ed 17, St Louis, 2003, Mosby.

MATCHING II

Match each term with the correct description.

1. _____ Is performed to remodel a previous scar or to remove a keloid.

2. _____ Is the removal of nonviable tissue from a nonhealing or traumatic wound.

3. _____ Is performed to replace skin that has been lost as a result of trauma, disease, or infection.

4. _____ Done to improve vision of the upper visual fields.

5. _____ Is performed to lift the supportive structures of the brow and alleviate drooping of skin, muscle, and fascia.

6. _____ Redundant and sagging supportive tissue of the face is reduced or modified to provide a more aesthetic appearance.

7. _____ Surgical creation of the external ear

8. _____ Is performed to increase the size and improve the shape of the breast.

9. _____ Is performed to reduce excess breast tissue.

10. _____ Transverse rectus abdominis myocutaneous flap

11. _____ Is performed to remove excess deep fat.

12. _____ Is performed to remove excess skin and adipose tissue from the abdominal wall.

a. Liposuction
b. Split-thickness skin graft
c. Augmentation mammoplasty
d. Scar revision
e. Otoplasty
f. Panniculectomy
g. Brow lift
h. Debridement of burns
i. TRAM
j. Blepharoplasty
k. Reduction mammoplasty
l. Rhytidectomy

CASE STUDIES

1. *Your patient is coming to surgery for debridement of a burn. Your knowledge of burns helps you choose the skin grafting instruments that will be needed. Describe the different types of burns listed below using the American Burn Association classification system.*

   a. Superficial partial-thickness, first-degree

b. Partial-thickness, second-degree

c. Full-thickness, second-degree

d. Full-thickness, third-degree

2. *Your patient has a congenital malformation of the external ear. What procedure would be used to correct this condition? What type of dressing would be used after this procedure?*

31 Orthopedic Surgery

Student's Name _____

KEY TERMS

Write the definition for each term.

1. Alloy: _____

2. Aponeurosis: _____

3. Arthrodesis: _____

4. Bioactive implant: _____

5. Biocompatibility: _____

6. Biomechanics: _____

7. Broaches: _____

8. Cannulated: _____

9. Casting: _____

10. Closed reduction: _____

11. Comminuted: _____

12. Compartment syndrome: _____

13. Compression: _____

14. Cruciate: _____

15. Dislocation: _____

16. Distraction: _____

17. Examination under anesthesia (EUA): _____

18. External fixation: _____

19. Internal fixation: _____

20. Open reduction: _____

21. Orthopedic system: _____

22. Press-fit: _____

23. Ream: _____

24. Replantation: _____

25. Reduction: _____

26. Skeletal traction: _____

27. Traction: _____

LABELING

Label this figure of the anatomy of a long bone using the descriptions and medical terminology as described in the text.

1. _____

2. _____

3. _____

4. _____

5. _____

6. _____

7. _____

8. _____

9. _____

10. _____

11. _____

12. _____

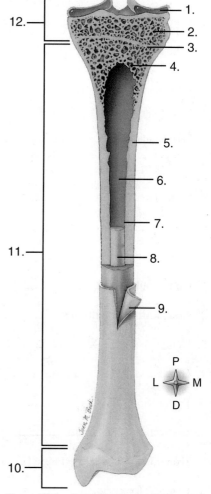

From Thibodeau G, Patton K: *Anatomy and physiology*, ed 6, St Louis, 2007, Mosby.

The figures below illustrate several types of orthopedic drills. Please label each illustration.

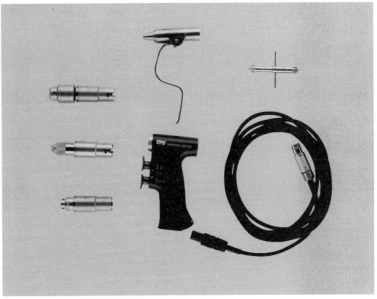

(From Tighe SM: *Instrumentation for the operating room*, ed 6, St Louis, 2003, Mosby.)

1. _____

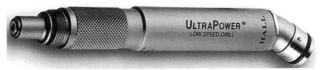

(Courtesy Zimmer, Warsaw, Ind.)

2. _____

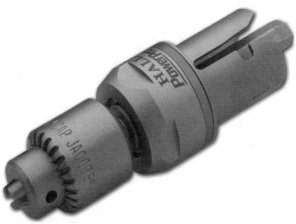

(Courtesy Zimmer, Warsaw, Ind.)

3. _____

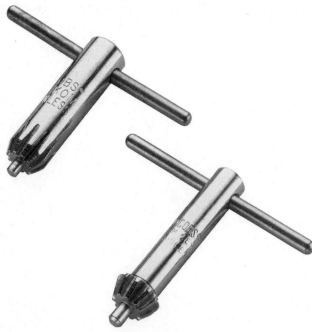

(Courtesy Zimmer, Warsaw, Ind.)

4. _____

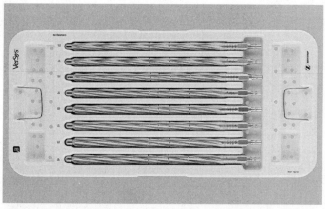

(From Tighe SM: *Instrumentation for the operating room*, ed 6, St Louis, 2003, Mosby.)

5. _____

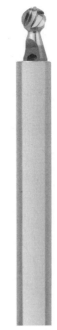

(Courtesy Zimmer, Warsaw, Ind.)

6. _____

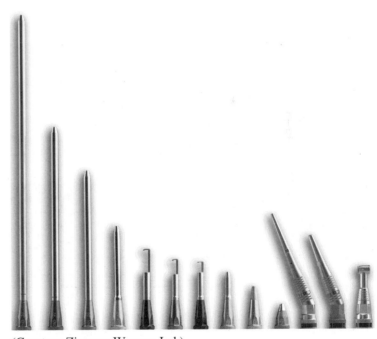

(Courtesy Zimmer, Warsaw, Ind.)

7. _____

Provide a short answer for each question or statement.

1. What are the three stages of bone healing, and what occurs during each phase?

    a. _____

    b. _____

    c. _____

2. How are joints classified?

    a. _____

    b. _____

    c. _____

3. List the equipment, supplies, and medication used in orthopedic surgery.

    _____

    _____

4. List the different types of instruments used in orthopedic surgery and give an example.

    _____

    _____

5. List the different types of fracture patterns and give an example of each.

    _____

    _____

6. List the different types of fracture repairs and define.

    _____

    _____

7. List the parts of a screw and define.

    _____

    _____

8. List and define the different types of screws.

_____

_____

9. List the functions of a plating system.

_____

_____

10. List and define the different types of plates.

_____

_____

11. Define and give an example of: IM rod, wires and cables, K-wires and Steinmann pins.

_____

_____

12. Traction is used for:

_____

_____

13. List and define the different types of metal used for joint replacement.

_____

_____

14. For which of the following medical diagnoses would the surgical intervention be arthroplasty? Write "arthroplasty" on the line if it would be used.

a. Avascular necrosis: _____

b. Rheumatoid arthritis: _____

c. Malignant bone tumor: _____

d. Metastatic bone disease: _____

e. Osteoporosis: _____

f. Scoliosis: _____

g. Compartment syndrome: _____

15. What imaging procedures are used to diagnose orthopedic trauma and disease?

MATCHING

1. _____ A ridge of bone

2. _____ A sharp, narrow projection

3. _____ A knuckle-shaped portion of bone, generally found in association with a joint

4. _____ A projection of bone

5. _____ A small, rounded projection

6. _____ A large, rounded projection

7. _____ A rounded orifice in bone, a passageway for blood vessels or nerves

8. _____ A cavity within a bone

9. _____ A groove in a bone

Match each medical term for these bone landmarks with the correct definition.

a. Sulcus

b. Crest

c. Condyle

d. Tubercle

e. Foramen

f. Sinus

g. Spine

h. Tuberosity

i. Process

1. *Your patient has just arrived in the emergency department with orthopedic trauma that resulted in possible vascular and spinal cord injuries. He will need to be evaluated and then diagnosed using a variety of imaging procedures. Which imaging techniques would be used to specifically diagnose the vascular and spinal cord injuries?*

   a.

   b.

2. *You have just been called in for orthopedic trauma. Knowing the types of bone fractures helps you choose the type of instrumentation needed for the repair. Working from left to right, label the fractures pictured in the following figure.*

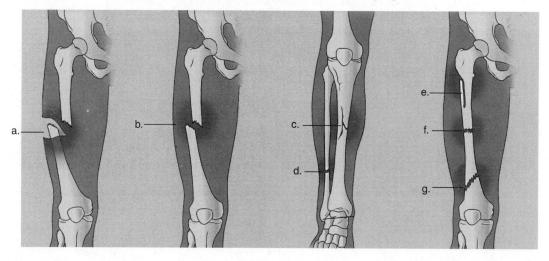

a.

b.

c.

d.

e.

f.

g.

32 Peripheral Vascular Surgery

Student's Name _____

KEY TERMS

Write the definition for each term.

1. Aneurysm: _____

2. Angioplasty: _____

3. Arteriosclerosis: _____

4. Arteriotomy: _____

5. Atherosclerosis: _____

6. Bifurcation: _____

7. Doppler duplex ultrasonography: _____

8. Embolus: _____

9. Endarterectomy: _____

10. Hemodialysis: _____

11. Hemodynamic: _____

12. In situ: _____

13. Infarction: _____

14. Intravascular ultrasound: _____

15. Ischemia: _____

16. Lumen: _____

17. Percutaneous: _____

18. Stent: _____

19. Thrombus: _____

20. Umbilical tape: _____

21. Venous stasis: _____

22. Vessel loop: _____

LABELING I

Label the pulmonary and systemic vascular circulation.

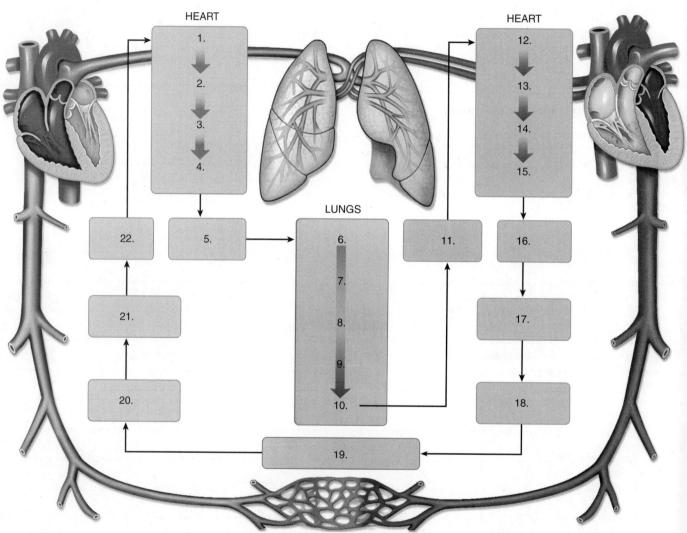

From Thibodeau G, Patton K: *Anatomy and physiology*, ed 6, St Louis, 2007, Mosby.

1. _____   5. _____

2. _____   6. _____

3. _____   7. _____

4. _____   8. _____

9. _____
10. _____
11. _____
12. _____
13. _____
14. _____
15. _____

16. _____
17. _____
18. _____
19. _____
20. _____
21. _____
22. _____

Working from left to right, label the vascular scissors shown.

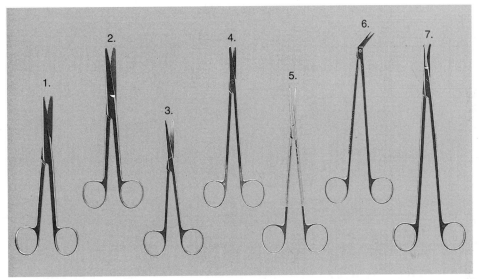

From Tighe SM: *Instrumentation for the operating room*, ed 7, St Louis, 2007, Mosby.

1. _____
2. _____
3. _____
4. _____

5. _____
6. _____
7. _____

SHORT ANSWER

Provide a short answer for each question or statement.

1. List the structures of the blood vessel and define.

   _____

   _____

2. Define blood pressure and list how normal blood pressure is affected:

   _____

   _____

3. List the blood vessels of the body and give an example of each:

   a. _____

   b. _____

   c. _____

   d. _____

   e. _____

   f. _____

   g. _____

   h. _____

4. List the diagnostic procedures associated with peripheral vascular surgery.

   a. _____

   b. _____

   c. _____

   d. _____

5. List and give an example of instruments used in peripheral vascular surgery.

   a. _____

   b. _____

   c. _____

   d. _____

f. After the case, what should you do?

2. *Patients with end-stage renal disease require frequent hemodialysis. This treatment requires long-term access to the patient's vascular system. What surgical interventions might be needed to create a means of long-term access?*

c. Will your patient need to go on bypass for the procedure?

2. *Why is a local anesthetic sprayed into the trachea (even if the patient is under general anesthesia) before the endoscope is inserted for a bronchoscopy?*

34 Cardiac Surgery

Student's Name _____

KEY TERMS

Write the definition for each term.

1. Aneurysm: _____

2. Apex: _____

3. Arrhythmia: _____

4. Arteriosclerosis: _____

5. Atherosclerosis: _____

6. Bradycardia: _____

7. Cardiac Cycle: _____

8. Cardioplegia: _____

9. Coarctation: _____

10. Congenital: _____

11. Cross-clamp: _____

12. Diastole: _____

13. Endovascular repair: _____

14. Fibrillation: _____

15. Fusiform aneurysm: _____

16. Heart lung machine: _____

17. Infarction: _____

18. Ischemia: _____

19. Off-pump procedure: _____

20. Pacemaker: _____

21. Preclotting: _____

22. Saccular aneurysm: _____

23. Shunt: _____

24. Stenosis: _____

25. Sternotomy: _____

26. Systole: _____

27. Tachycardia: _____

28. Thoracotomy: _____

LABELING

Using the following diagram, label the components of the conduction system of the heart.

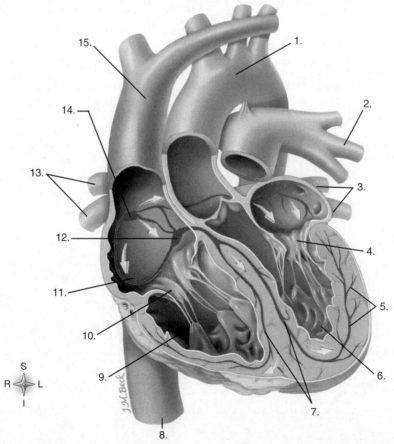

Modified from Thibodeau G, Patton K: *Anatomy and physiology,* ed 6, St Louis, 2007, Mosby.

1. _____   3. _____

2. _____   4. _____

5. _____   11. _____

6. _____   12. _____

7. _____   13. _____

8. _____   14. _____

9. _____   15. _____

10. _____

SHORT ANSWER

Provide a short answer for each question or statement.

1. What structures are in the thoracic cavity?

   _____

   _____

2. List the diagnostic tests associated with cardiac surgery.

   _____

   _____

3. List the equipment, supplies, and medication associated with cardiac surgery.

   _____

   _____

4. List the different types of instruments associated with cardiac surgery.

   _____

   _____

5. Define the following surgical procedures:

   a. Cardiac catheterization

   _____

   _____

   b. Vessel and patch grafts

   _____

   _____

307

c. Prosthetic valves

_____

_____

d. Pacemaker

_____

_____

e. Cardiopulmonary bypass

_____

_____

f. Median sternotomy

_____

_____

g. Sump catheterization

_____

_____

h. CABG

_____

_____

i. Transmyocardial revascularization

_____

_____

j. Resection of a left ventricular aneurysm

_____

_____

k. Aortic valve replacement

_____

_____

l. Mitral valve repair and replacement

_____

_____

m. Resection of an aneurysm of the ascending aorta

_____

_____

n. Resection of an aneurysm of the ascending arch

_____

_____

o. Resection of an aneurysm of the descending thoracic aorta

_____

_____

p. Endovascular repair of a thoracic aneurysm

_____

_____

q. Insertion of an artificial cardiac pacemaker

_____

_____

r. Temporary pacemaker

_____

_____

s. Epicardial pacemaker

_____

_____

t. Replacement of a pacemaker battery

_____

_____

u. Implantable cardioverter defibrillator

_____

_____

v. Surgery for atrial fibrillation

_____

_____

w. Pericardial window

_____

_____

x. Pericardiectomy

_____

_____

y. Insertion and removal of an intraaortic balloon catheter

_____

_____

z. Ventricular assist device

_____

_____

aa. Heart transplantation

_____

_____

MATCHING

Match each term with the correct definition.

1. _____ Weakening of the heart muscle caused by obstruction of coronary arteries

2. _____ Cause of CAD

3. _____ Condition in which the heart cells quiver rather than contract effectively

4. _____ Type of hardening of the arteries that results in stiffness and loss of function

5. _____ Weakening of the wall of an artery or the heart chamber, leading to thinning and ballooning

6. _____ Cause for this would include valve disease

7. _____ Excess fluid in the pericardium

8. _____ Chronic inflammation of the pericardium

9. _____ Heart rate below 60 beats/min

10. _____ Possible narrowing of aortic and mitral valve or valves

11. _____ Cardiac muscle that beats abnormally fast

12. _____ Immune-mediated disease

a. Aneurysm
b. Arteriosclerosis
c. Atrial fibrillation
d. Bradycardia
e. Heart transplantation
f. Atherosclerosis
g. Myocardial Infarction
h. Pericardial effusion
i. Pericarditis
j. Rheumatic heart disease
k. Valve stenosis
l. Tachycardia

CASE STUDIES

1. _Your patient has just had a heart attack and is asking about the term cardiac cycle. How would you explain the cardiac cycle to your patient?_

35 Pediatric Surgery

Student's Name _____

Write the definition for each term.

1. Acquired anomaly: _____

2. Atresia: _____

3. Bolus: _____

4. Child life specialist: _____

5. Choanal: _____

6. Coarctation: _____

7. Congenital: _____

8. Ductus arteriosus: _____

9. Embryonic life: _____

10. Exstrophy: _____

11. Fetus: _____

12. Genetic abnormality: _____

13. Homeostasis: _____

14. Isolette: _____

15. Magical thinking: _____

16. Mutagenic substance: _____

17. Nephroblastoma: _____

18. Neutral tube defect: _____

19. Omphalocele: _____

20. Pyloric stenosis: _____

21. Teratogen: _____

SHORT ANSWERS

Provide a short answer for each question or statement.

1. Name three interventions used to keep pediatric patients warm in surgery.

   a. _____

   b. _____

   c. _____

2. What is the surgical technologist's responsibility in reporting and calculating blood loss in pediatric patients?

   _____

   _____

3. Babies with esophageal atresia or a transesophageal fistula usually are low-birth-weight babies. Why?

   _____

   _____

4. What is Hirschsprung disease?

   _____

   _____

5. What is epispadias?

   _____

   _____

6. Coarctation of the thoracic aorta is a congenital stenosis. What does correction of this congenital condition do for the patient?

   _____

   _____

7. What are the specific defects in tetralogy of Fallot?

   _____

   _____

8. What is the primary differences regarding electrosurgery in the pediatric patient versus the adult patient?

_____

_____

9. List the equipment, supplies, and medication related to pediatric surgery.

_____

_____

10. List the specialty instrumentation related to pediatric surgery.

_____

_____

11. Thermoregulation is important during pediatric surgery. List and define the two risks that pediatric patients are particularly vulnerable to.

_____

_____

12. What should the room temperature be for pediatric surgery?

_____

_____

13. List the interventions during pediatric surgery to maintain normothermia.

_____

_____

14. List the steps of case planning and give an example of each.

_____

_____

15. List the developmental stages of the child and list a psychological characteristic.

_____

_____

16. List the safety of the pediatric patient during:

a. Safe handling of drugs:

_____

_____

b. Transportation

_____

_____

c. Positioning

_____

_____

d. Electrosurgery

_____

_____

e. Instruments

_____

_____

f. Sponges

_____

_____

g. Sutures

_____

_____

17. Define the following surgical procedures:

a. Repair of a cleft lip

_____

_____

b. Repair of a cleft palate

_____

_____

c. Otoplasty

_____

_____

d. Reconstruction of the ear

_____

_____

e. Pyloromyotomy

_____

_____

f. Resection and pull-through for Hirschsprung disease

_____

_____

g. Bowel reconstruction for imperforate anus

_____

_____

h. Reduction of an intussusception

_____

_____

i. Reduction of a volvulus

_____

_____

j. Closure of an atrial septal defect

_____

_____

k. Closure of an ventricular septal defect

_____

_____

l. Repair of rectus excavatum

_____

_____

m. Nephrectomy in Wilms tumor

_____

_____

n. Repair of myelomeningocele

_____

_____

o. Correction of syndactyly

_____

_____

MATCHING

Match each medical diagnosis with the correct definition.

1. _____ Absence or closure of an orifice or a tubular structure

2. _____ Narrowing of the passageway of a blood vessel, such as coarctation of the aorta

3. _____ Eversion or turning out of an organ

4. _____ Herniation of abdominal contents through the abdominal wall, present at birth

5. _____ Telescoping of one portion of the intestine into another

6. _____ Wilms tumor

7. _____ Congenital abnormality resulting from failure of the neural tube to close in embryonic development

8. _____ Protrusion of abdominal contents through an opening at the navel, especially when occurring as a congenital defect

9. _____ Narrowing of the part of the stomach (pylorus) that leads to the small intestines

a. Pyloric stenosis

b. Exstrophy

c. Coarctation

d. Atresia

e. Omphalocele

f. Neural tube defect

g. Gastroschisis

h. Nephroblastoma

i. Intussusception

CASE STUDIES

1. *Some things both in the environment and in the diet of a pregnant woman are teratogenic to the fetus. What are they?*

2. *You are called in on call to do an exploratory laparotomy. Your patient is 2 hours old.*

   a. What supplies and equipment will you need?

   b. What special equipment would you use?

b. What procedure will the surgeon suggest to the patient as a potential cure?

c. How will the surgeon describe to the patient the potential postoperative complications for this procedure?

d. Where will the incision be?

2. *Your surgical case today is an open craniotomy for removal of a tumor. The surgeon is going to "turn a flap," including the bone. As the scrub, what is your responsibility with regard to the bone if it is removed from the patient?*

37 Emergency Trauma Surgery

Student's Name _____

KEY TERMS

Write the definition for each term.

1. Advance Trauma Life Support (ATLS): _____

2. Algorithms: _____

3. Blunt injury: _____

4. Cardiac rupture: _____

5. Cardiac tamponade: _____

6. Coagulopathy: _____

7. Compartment syndrome: _____

8. Contusions: _____

9. Damage control surgery: _____

10. Definitive diagnosis: _____

11. Definitive procedure: _____

12. Exsanguinating: _____

13. Flail chest: _____

14. Focused assessment with ultrasound for trauma (FAST): _____

15. Hemorrhagic shock: _____

16. Hemothorax: _____

17. Metabolic acidosis: _____

18. Occult injury: _____

19. Penetrating injury: _____

20. Pneumothorax: _____

21. Resuscitation: _____

SHORT ANSWER

Provide a short answer for each question or statement.

1. List the diagnostic tests associated with a trauma.

   _____

   _____

2. List the equipment, supplies, and medication associated with a trauma.

   _____

   _____

3. List the specialty instruments that might be used in a trauma case.

   _____

   _____

4. List the trauma system and define.

   _____

   _____

5. List and define the lethal triad.

   _____

   _____

6. List the ATLS principles of trauma management.

   _____

   _____

7. List and define the primary and secondary survey.

   _____

   _____

8. List and give an example of the preoperative care of the patient.

   _____

   _____

9. List the proper way to manage the sterile field in an emergency trauma.

_____

_____

10. List and give an example of the following surgical procedures related to trauma:

    a. Laparotomy with staged closure

_____

_____

    b. Abdominal trauma

_____

_____

    c. Abdominal compartment syndrome

_____

_____

    d. Orthopedic trauma

_____

_____

    e. Orthopedic fractures

_____

_____

    f. Thoracic injury

_____

_____

    g. Cardiovascular trauma

_____

_____

h. Penetrating cardiac wound

_____

_____

i. Flail chest

_____

_____

j. Aortic injury

_____

_____

k. Hemothorax

_____

_____

l. Laceration of the lung

_____

_____

m. Trauma of the brain and spinal cord

_____

_____

n. Trauma related to major peripheral vascular trauma

_____

_____

CHART COMPLETION

Complete the following chart:

Techniques for Temporary Abdominal Closure

Technique	Description	Mechanism
1. _____	A perforated plastic sheet covers the viscera, and a sponge is placed between the fascial edges. The wound is covered by an airtight seal, which is pierced by a suction drain connected to a suction pump and fluid collection system.	The (active and adjustable) negative pressure supplied by the pump keeps constant tension on the fascial edges while it collects excess abdominal fluid and helps resolve edema.
2. _____	A perforated plastic sheet covers the viscera, damp surgical towels are placed in the wound, and a surgical drain is placed on the towels. An air-tight seal covers the wound, and negative pressure is applied through the drain.	The negative pressure keeps constant tension on the fascial edges, and excess fluid is collected.
3. _____	Two opposite Velcro sheets (hooks and loops, one on each side) are sutured to the fascial edges. The Velcro sheets connect in the middle.	This technique allows for easy access and stepwise reapproximation of the fascial edges.
4. _____	The viscera are covered with a sheet (e.g., ISODrape, Microtek [Microban], Huntersville, NC). Horizontal sutures are placed through a large-diameter catheter and through the entire abdominal wall on both sides.	The sutures keep tension on the fascia and may be tightened to allow staged reapproximation of the fascial edges. This may be combined with a vacuum system.
5. _____	A sterile x-ray film cassette bag or sterile 3-L urology irrigation bag is sutured between the fascial edges or the skin and opened in the middle.	This is an easy technique that allows for easy access. The bag may be reduced in size to approximate the fascial edges.
6. _____	An absorbable or nonabsorbable mesh or sheet is sutured between the fascial edges. Examples are Dexon, Marlex, or Vicryl mesh. Examples of sheets are Silastic or silicone sheets.	The mesh or sheet may be reduced in size to allow for reapproximation. Nonresorbable meshes may be removed or left in place at the end of the open abdominal period.

Modified from Diaz J, Duton W, Miller R: The difficult abdominal wall. In Townsend CM Jr, Beauchamp RD, Evers BM, Mattox KL, editors: *Sabiston textbook of surgery*, ed 19, Philadelphia, 2012, WB Saunders.

1. *You are called in for a stab wound to the thoracic cavity.*

    a. What type of instruments would you need?

    b. What hemostatic agents would need?

    c. What specialty instruments would you need?

    d. What equipment would you need?

    e. What type of retractor would you need?

2. *You are called in for an gunshot to the right femur, the patient has a shattered femur and there is vascular damage.*

    a. What type of instruments would you need?

    b. What hemostatic agents would need?

    c. What specialty instruments would you need?

    d. What equipment would you need?

    e. What type of retractor would you need?